Cover Design and Artwork	:	**Blazon Business Outsourcing(BBO)**
Published by	:	**M&A Resource Training and Publishing Inc.**
Website	:	**www.matrainingcenter.com**

Printed in the Philippines
ISBN 971-92605-1-3

Previously Published as "In-House Doctor" First Printing	- 2003
E-book Publication	- 2013

In an effort to support local communities, raise awareness and funds, M&A Resource Training and Publishing Inc. donates a percentage of sales of each book to WordSpring Foundation Inc. and Oro Investment and Microfinance Cooperative.

Foreword

I met Dr. Edward Cagape on a warm summer night in Davao City, on the island of Mindanao, Philippines. I was sitting across a table filled with delicious Filipino dishes cooked by his wife, Cora. Dr. Cagape is not your typical heart surgeon. He is passionate about helping his patients, and anyone who needs medical care wherever they are. He is easy to talk with; full of humor as he regales me with tales of his life and hilarious incidents.

I went to Davao to get to know Dr. Cagape at the request of his sister Rosemarie, whom I met at my Rotary Club in Dallas, Texas, USA. Other than his sister, I really had no agenda or reason to be there. Part way through the meal, Dr. Cagape asked me what I do for a living. When he found out that I had a publishing company in the US, he got up to get something to show me: a copy of his book entitled, "In-House Doctor".

The early edition of the book that Dr. Cagape brought us both to start on a journey that has ended with you holding and reading this completely revised edition; "Self-Medical Diagnosis". It has been published in the Philippines, not only because of the great need for it there, but also to bypass the need for endless legal considerations and consultations that would have been required in the US!

Medical Care is increasingly one of the most crucial needs of humankind. As the world population grows, depleted lands produce less nutrition, and chemicals and the side effects of technology create stress and health complications; any spark of hope becomes a beacon in the darkness. This book will be that spark of hope for many.

Why publish information that until now has only been entrusted to fully-degreed and licensed physicians? Are there no dangers in allowing the untrained minds to have access to this? Making this information public may be controversial to some, but to the many who are far from medical care, either physically or financially, this information is timely. Even as a way to get a second opinion, this is a valuable tool to anyone who can barely afford to see even a physician, not to mention the doubled expense for a second opinion.

A few weeks ago I read a news article that Michael Bloomberg, the Mayor of New York City, has banned food donations to homeless shelters, because the city can't assess their salt, fat and fiber content. Most people sadly shake their head over the lack of logical thinking on decisions of that type. I'm sure many a hungry homeless person living on the streets would benefit much more in their quality of life by eating a meal, that perhaps, had more fat or salt than the city recommends.

In the same way, I would much rather see a person with a life threatening condition discover in this book that they have a serious condition, and get treatment for it, than, continue to their death, not knowing that their symptoms were much more serious than they imagined.

Thank you for considering this essential guide. If you have family, church members, or anyone you know who needs this book, please consider obtaining another copy to give to them. If we all work together, we can improve the quality of health in our community.

To Your Health,

Bob Bare
Chairman
M&A Resource Training and Publishing Inc.

PREFACE

The purpose of this book is for the layman to understand the basic elements of self-medication. This covers a whole range of the causes of pains, the different diseases and the prescribed medicines that could be used to temporarily alleviate the pain.

Likewise, it teaches the layman to decide whether there is a need for a medical checkup, to understand physician's recommendation such as diagnostic work–up and the complications of an illness that may result without proper action. This book is a good avenue in taking care of his or her own health and to have the freedom and the confidence to decide which is best for one's own health.

At a time, when we are bombarded with thousands of recommendations, each one claiming to have the best cure it the traditional medicines of the East, Indian herbal medications, homoeopathy, local barrio treatments, health supplements from different multivitamin companies, etc. - an individual can be confused of what to do with his or her ailment. More often than not, he or she tends to experiment just to have a sigh of relief from said illness.

This book tries to explain in laymen's term the anatomical basis of illnesses: what to do with them and how to deal with them properly. Moreover, it corrects superstitious techniques in handling illnesses that are believed to be the perfect way in curing them.

This book does not attempt to cover all illnesses that we have today. However, the most common illnesses are discussed inside these chapters and the reader is recommended to search for answers in other areas of medical science to satisfy their curiosity.

Your neighbor's expert advice, regarding his personal experience of a particular sickness does not apply to you. More so, if he is not a doctor. There are thousands of symptoms that lead to thousands diagnoses. Whatever happened to your neighbor and how he was able to survive is only one of several methods used to fight or cure a disease. You are unique and different.

Medicine has come a long way. It has done away with thousand and different medical managements that are not repeatable (read: bad results, good results but not lasting, bad results with good endings, good results but patient is scarred, etc.)

It has streamlined its management of illness. Protocols have been made to suit which medicine is good for what illness. Backed up by several thousand trials, followed up with millions of patient care, the doctor has the last say in the management of diseases. It's not your nosy neighbor or the salesman who sells you all those health enhancers and vitamins nor the advertisements you read in the news that will make the therapeutic supervision.

The only problem with doctors is that they don't speak your language. You want to know what is happening to you but they cannot explain it to you in simple terms.

This books bridges this gap of communication. Common illnesses are explained to you in simple terms. And this book goes further.

Through this book you will know what ails you long before your doctor examines you. You can practically "walk" the diagnosis with him. Decide whether the laboratory exams he is doing on you follows the diagnosis he is saying; decide for yourself whether you will go on with the diagnostics or find another doctor. By reading this book, you will not be groping in the dark while having the feeling of being the "guinea pig". This time, you become a participant in the quest for answers with your doctor.

After all the lab exams have been done and you are given the option to be operated or not, you should know what will be done to you; what are the complications if surgery will be conducted and the possible results if you will not undergo surgery.

Finally, this book enables the layman to understand his or her doctor much better than before. It was never the intention of this book to make anyone a doctor or better than the doctor.

Edward R. Cagape, MD

ACKNOWLEDGEMENTS:

I would like to acknowledge all the websites I have visited and have in one way or the other helped me in completing this book, most especially, the following:

http://www.diabetes.org

http://www.HealthCenter.com

http://www.lungusa.org

http://www.Medlineplus.gov

http://www.commoncold.org

http://www.familydoctor.org

http://www.mesothelioma-facts.com

http://www.spinalinjury.net

http://www.virtualhospital.com

http://www.nyerrn.com

Prostate Cancer Institute

Electronic Textbook of Dermatology

DEDICATION

This revised version, like the first book is dedicated to the following: to the common people who want to understand why they are sick; to people who need a doctor in the middle of the night; to those who do not have access to a doctor either physically and financially; and to those who want to understand their doctor better and desire to "walk through" the diagnoses with them.

Finally, this book is dedicated to my beautiful wife Cora who has blessed me with four amazing children, namely: Edward, Lady Magaret, Rajiv and Emmanuel.

Dr. Edward Cagape

TABLE OF CONTENTS

FOREWORD i

PREFACE iii

ACKNOWLEDGEMENTS v

DEDICATION vi

CHAPTER 1 (Bodily Pains) 1

ABDOMINAL PAIN 2

    Epigastric Pain.. 3

    Epigastric Pains + Nonhealing Ulcer 5

    Epigastric Pains + Right Lower Quadrant Pain.. 7

    Epigastric Pain + Loose Bowel Movement 9

    Epigastric Pain + Chest Pain 11

    Epigastric Pain + Right or Left Flank Pain... 13

    Right Upper Quadrant Pain 16

    Right Upper Quadrant Pain + Yellow Discoloration of the Eyes.. 18

    Hypogastric Pains + Frequency of Urination 21

    Left Lower Quadrant Pain in the Adult... 23

    Left Lower Quadrant Pain in the Young 25

    Whole Abdominal Pain in Children + No Bowel Movement for 24 Hrs 27

    Hypogastric Pains + Vaginal Spotting 29

    Hypogastric Pains + Menstruation... 30

    Right Inguinal Pain (or Left) + Mass in the Scrotum.. 32

    Right or Left Flank Pain 34

    SCROTAL PAINS.. 36

    Pain in the Scrotum In Mumps... 38

    Pain in the Scrotum In Varicocele 40

    Pain in the Scrotum In Testicular Torsion.. 41

    PAINS OF THE CHEST AND BREAST PAINS.. 42

    Chest Pain + Numbness of Left Arm... 43

    Chest Pains + Hyperacidity.. 45

    Chest Pain + Pain on Inspiration 46

    Chest Pain + Cough 48

    Chest Pain + Vesicle Formation... 50

    Breast Pain in 18 Yr Old.. 51

Breast Pain in 25 Yr Old Single 52

Breast Pain During Lactation 53

Breast Pain During Menopause 54

Breast Pain + A Mass in An 18 Yr Old 55

Breast Pain + Round Mass in a 21 Yr Old 56

Breast Pain + Mass in a 35 Yr Old 54

Breast Pain + Nipple Discharge (Bloody) in a 25 Yr Old 57

HEADACHES 61

Frontal Headache 62

Migraine Headache 64

Stress Pains 66

Preauricular Pain 67

Nuchal Pain 69

Occipital Pain 70

Generalized Headache 72

Postauricular Pain 74

Infra-auricular Pain 75

EXTREMITY PAINS AND NUMBNESS 77

Joint Pains 78

Tennis Elbow 80

Pain and Numbness of the Upper Extremity 82

Sciatica 84

ANAL PAINS 86

Anal Pain after Constipation 87

Pain at the Anal Side 88

Anal Pain + Bleeding + Constipation 90

Anal Pain in Hemorrhoids 92

BACK PAINS 95

Interscapular Pains 96

Torticulis 98

Back Pain + Cough +Smoking 99

Back Pain + History of TB 101

Low Back Pains 103

Low Back Pains + Shooting Pains to the Legs 105

PAIN DURING URINATION 107

   Pain During Urination without Discharge 109

PAIN IN THE NECK DURING SWALLOWING 110

   Sore Throat... 112

   Sore Throat + Colds 113

   Sore Throat + Acute Hoarseness 114

   Sore Throat + Chronic Hoarseness 116

   Difficulty of Swallowing + Fever 117

   Difficulty of Swallowing + No Fever 119

   Swallowed Coins 120

PAIN IN THE EAR... 122

   Pain in the Ear + Fullness 123

   Pain in the Ear + Itchiness 124

CHAPTER 2 (Reddening And Wounds) **126**

REDDENING AND DARK

DISCOLORATIONS OF THE SKIN.. 128

   Trauma... 129

   Hematoma 130

   Insect Bite... 132

   Skin Infection 134

   Abscess 135

   Furunculosis 137

   Infected Sebaceous Cyst... 139

   Dark Discoloration of the Skin.. 141

   Cat Bite.. 143

   Dog Bite... 144

   Insect Bite... 146

   Rat Bite.. 147

   Human Bite 148

   Superficial Wounds 150

   Skin Abscess without Opening 152

   Skin Abscess with Pustule... 154

   Skin Ulceration 155

   Wounds and Blunt Injury to the Chest 157

Wounds and Blunt Injury to the Abdomen 159

Wounds and Blunt Injury to the Neck 161

Wounds of the Face 163

BLOOD IN URINE 164

Blood in the Urine + Pain in the Flanks 166

Bloody Urine + Pain Inguinal and Scrotum (Male) 168

Bloody Urine + Frequency o f Urination 170

Bloody Urine + No Urinary Stream Force 172

BLOOD IN THE SPUTUM 174

Bloody Sputum + Cough + Afternoon Fever 175

Bloody Sputum + Lost of Weight + Chest Pains 176

Bloody Sputum + Severe Forceful Cough 178

VOMITING BLOOD (HEMATEMESIS) 180

Drunk Severe Vomiting Blood 182

NOSE BLEEDING 184

BLOOD IN ANUS AND STOOLS 186

Fresh Blood from the Anus 187

Fresh Blood in the Anus + Abdominal Pain 188

Drops of Blood in Toilet Bowl 190

CHAPTER 3 (Fever) 182

F E V E R 193

Afternoon Fever 194

Fever with Chills 195

Fever + Watery Stools + Headache 196

Fever + Rashes on Legs 198

Fever + Cold + Cough 200

Fever + Yellowish 202

Fever + Jaundice + Abdominal Pain + Chills 204

Fever + Cough + Difficulty of Breathing 205

CHAPTER 4 (Difficulty of Body Movement) 207

FUNCTIO LAETIA 208

PARALYSIS 209

Paralysis Due to Stroke 210

Paralysis Due to Trauma to the Head 212

Paralysis Due to Brain Tumor 213

Paralysis After Back Bone Injury 214

Fractures 217

CHAPTER 5 (Difficulty of Breathing) **218**

DIFFICULTY OF BREATHING **219**

CHAPTER 6 (Cysts and cancer) **222**

Breast Cysts and Cancer 223

Tumors and Cancers of the Intestine 226

Tumors of the liver 229

Cancer of the Lungs 231

Tumors of the Uterus 233

Tumor of the Brain 235

Cancer of the Throat 237

Cysts and Cancer of the Skin 238

Enlargement of the Neck 241

Mass in the Anterior Neck 244

Mass above the Adam's Apple 246

Mass under the Mandible 248

Masses at the Side of the Neck 249

Mass Base of the Neck 251

Mass on the Side of the Neck 253

CHAPTER 7(Hypertension) **255**

Causes of Hypertension 256

Complications of Hypertension 257

Anti – Hypertension and Some of the Side Effects 258

CHAPTER 8 (Diabetes Mellitus) **260**

Diabetes Mellitus 261

Complications of Diabetes 262

CHAPTER 9 (Smoking) **265**

SMOKING *266*

The Normal Lung 267

The Smoker's Lung 268

The Heart In a Smoker 268

The Liver of the Smoker 269

The Legs and Toes of a Smoker 270

CHAPTER 10 (Stool Characteristics in Loose Bowel Movement) **271**

Fecal Characteristics 272

CHAPTER 11 (Emergency Procedures) **273**

Emergency Procedures: What You Can Do 274

Loss of Consciousness 274

Stabbed Wounds and Gun Shots Wounds 277

Burns 279

Choking 280

CHAPTER 12 (WOUND CARE) **281**

After Minor Operation 282

INDEX OF DIAGNOSIS 284

INDEX OF SURGICAL PROCEDURES 293

INDEX 301

HOW TO USE THIS BOOK

If you know the *symptoms* (i.e. abdominal pain):

1. Go to the main division dealing with the problem (DO – LOR – pains).
2. Look for the chapter dealing on the specific location of the problem (abdominal pains).
3. Find the schematic drawing pinpointing the location of the pain.

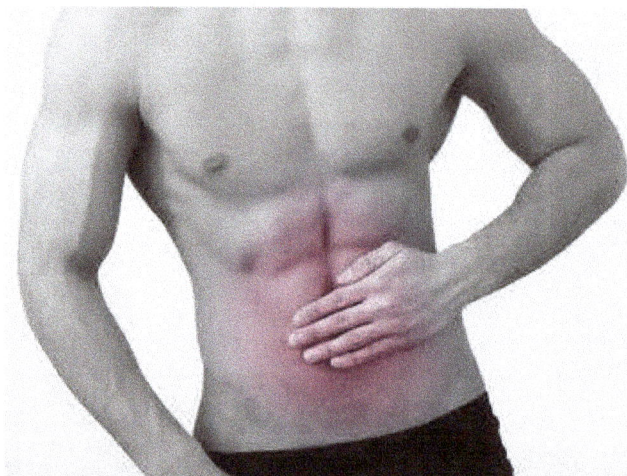

4. Determine the accompanying symptoms whether they match the symptoms you know (at least, 80% of the symptoms, because not all symptoms are always present as no single disease follows the same symptoms all the time).
5. Read the other diagnosis to confirm the similarity of the symptoms.
6. Obtain the diagnosis, initial treatment, laboratory exams and definitive treatments.

If you know the *diagnosis* given by your doctor i.e. FIBROCYSTIC DISEASE OF THE BREAST, the following steps are in order, namely:

1) You want to know what it is:

a) Go to Index at the back.

b) Find the page dealing with it.

c) Read the Foreword.

d) Look for the schematic drawing pinpointing the symptom.

e) Decide whether the diagnosis match the symptoms of your patient.

2) You want to know how it will be confirmed:

a) Read the laboratory exams and the DEFINITIVE TREATMENT expected to be done.

b) Discuss intelligently with your doctor what his management plan is and decide whether you got the best doctor for your patient (with you as his patient).

Chapter One

Bodily Pains

ABDOMINAL PAIN

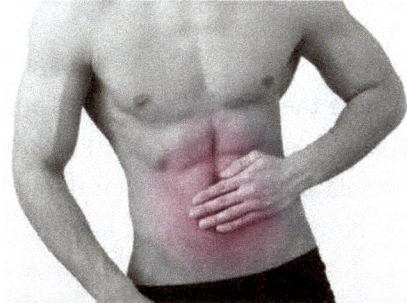

This chapter will deal on specific pains in the abdomen and their associated signs and symptoms.

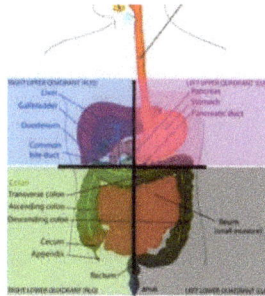

An abdominal pain that is felt in different areas pinpoints which internal organ is affected. For every abdominal pain, a specific disease is presented. Following this chapter, therefore, a layman who wants to know where the pain has started and where it radiates, would be given a hint as to what ails him. He will be given corresponding advice of what to do, whether to see a doctor immediately or to self-medicate, thereby, foregoing any further expense.

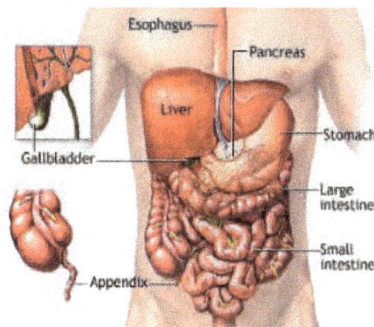

The reader must follow his or her own symptoms as they appear in chronological order. For example: abdominal pain is followed by nausea, then vomiting, then fever, then, the pain transfers to the right lower quadrant equals ACUTE APPENDICITIS.

Also, the reader must pinpoint where the pain is first located and go to the location indicated in the illustration. Read the description that would lead to A MOST PROBABLE diagnosis and the subsequent treatments. Accompanying symptoms should be taken into consideration to arrive in a definite diagnosis. However, there are lots of illnesses that do not have specific locations and therefore consultation with a surgeon is a must.

EPIGASTRIC PAIN

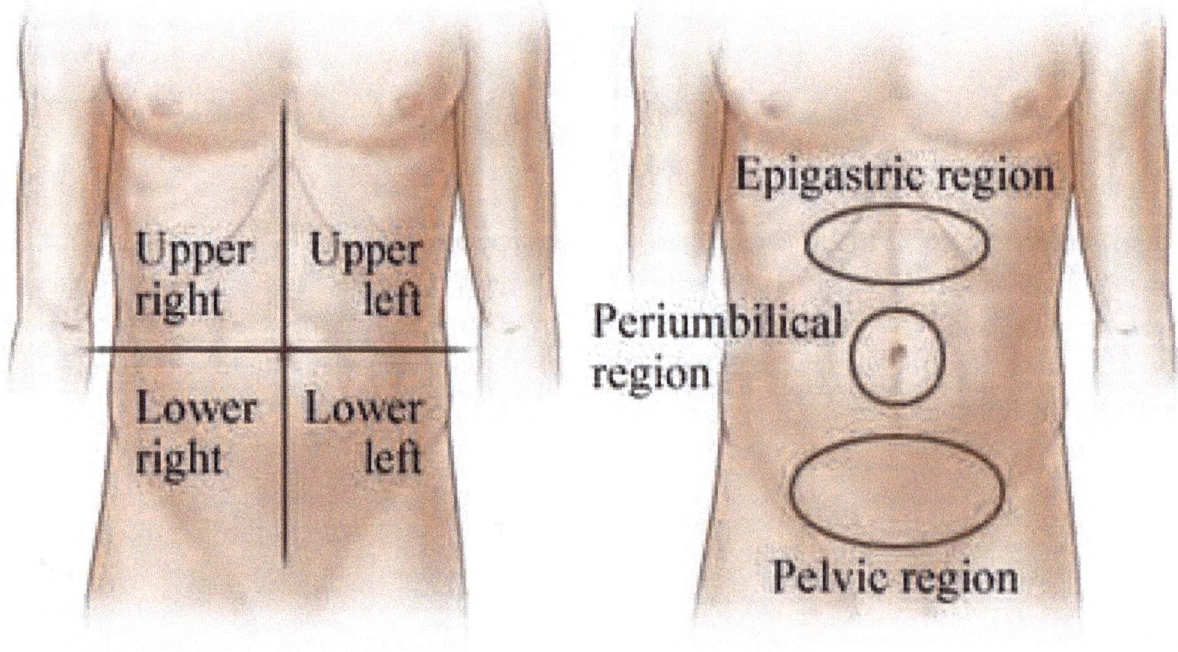

Epigastric pains that occur early in the morning, before breakfast and after meals are relieved by food intake or aggravated by hunger pangs. Some people would also feel back pain opposite to the location of epigastric pains.

(POSSIBLE)DIAGNOSIS: Peptic Ulcer
ORGAN INVOLVED: stomach
CAUSE: H. pylori

This can be caused by bacteria that actually erode the gastric mucosa or enhance ulcer formation. STRESS could also be a factor. Food is not known to directly cause the ulcer.

INITIAL TREATMENT: Any antacid

Kremil – S- 1 tab one hour after meal or **NOVALUZID** 1 sachet one hour after meal.

ADVICE:

Consultation with the doctor is needed to verify the extent of ulcer, duration of treatment and to differentiate from malignancy. (Whether said ulcer is malignant or not)

LABORATORY EXAM:

UPPER GI SERIES - a special kind of x-ray wherein the patient is asked to drink milk – like substance after which an x-ray of the abdomen is done. The patient is asked not to eat anything starting midnight up to the time of x-ray. X-ray films are taken in different position. Likewise, the patient is asked to lie flat, prone, and sideways in the dark room. All clothing will be taken off and a hospital gown is used during the procedure.

GASTROSCOPY - a special procedure wherein a very thin tube with a light on the tip (fiber - optic) is inserted inside the mouth down to the stomach to visualize the ulcer. The patient must not eat anything in the morning until the exam is done. The result can be seen on TV monitor and a direct biopsy (a piece of the stomach is taken) can be done subsequently. The procedure may trigger wreathing.

H. PYLORI DETERMINATION - blood exam to determine if H. pylori (A kind of bacteria responsible for causing peptic ulcer) is present.

OTHER DIAGNOSTIC MODALITIES: CT SCAN can be helpful if suspicion of cancer is present. MRI does not help and so is Ultrasound. This procedure cannot be diagnosed by any other lab exams.

DEFINITIVE TREATMENT:

H^2**BLOCKERS:** *PANTOPRAZOLE* 20 mg 1 tab daily for 45 days PLUS *AMOXYCILLIN* 500 mg 1 cap daily for 45 days.

EPIGASTRIC PAINS + NONHEALING ULCER

Chronic long standing pain in the upper portion of the abdomen with associated loss of weight, non-healing ulcer (for which no relief of pain even with the application of antacids and other ulcer medication) can be due to epigastric pain. A mass could be palpable in some cases. Tenderness can be felt when deep palpation is done in the epigastrium. Nausea and vomiting may occur due to obstruction of the outlet of the stomach. Early satiety may also occur.

DIAGNOSIS: GASTRIC MALIGNANCY

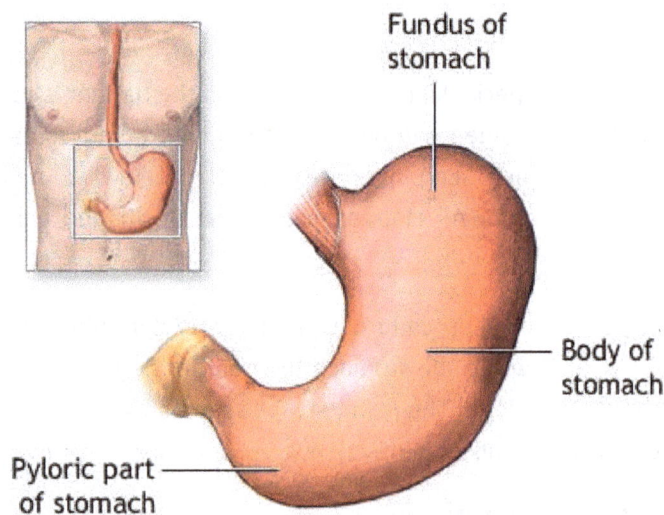

Fundus of stomach

Body of stomach

Pyloric part of stomach

ORGAN INVOLVED: Stomach

CAUSE: While the cause is *unknown, h*eredity is (can be) a factor, as well as, eating a lot of spicy and grilled foods.

INITIAL TREATMENT:
PAIN
> TRAMADOL 50 – 100 mg tablet every 6 hrs. **OR**
> BUSCOPAN tablet every 4 hrs. **OR** Hyoscine butylbromide
> BARALGIN tablet every 4 hrs.

VOMITING – small, frequent eating may help.

ADVICE: Long survival has been noted in cases early detected. Surgery is the major mode of treatment. (It has been noted that in cases which are detected, the patient has a long period of survival)

Modalities of adjuvant treatment like chemotherapy and radiotherapy also help in prolonging survival for more than five years.

LABORATORY EXAMINATIONS:

GASTROSCOPY + BIOPSY - a long fiber optic tube is inserted (inside) through the mouth (up until) into the stomach (to visualize) visualizing the tumor or ulcer. Biopsy of the suspected area is done to confirm the diagnosis.

UPPER GI SERIES - a series of x-ray examinations with the use of contrast media is used to visualize a mass in the stomach. Patient is asked to drink milk – like substance before the x-ray examination.

DEFINITIVE TREATMENT:

GASTRECTOMY – removal of the stomach (partial or total) with the intention of removing the whole tumor and its surrounding tissues. Continuity of the GASTROINTESTINAL TRACT is done through creation of a new stomach coming from a portion of the small intestine.

EPIGASTRIC PAINS + RIGHT LOWER QUADRANT PAIN

This is the pain that starts at the epigastric area then transfers to the right side of the abdomen followed by nausea, vomiting, and fever. No loose bowel movement is noted. Symptoms may vary from one person to another. Some patients do not have fever before the onset of right lower quadrant pain. Others do not have (experience) vomiting. Pain is not relieved by any position nor any antispasmodic or analgesic. Some would feel fullness or bloating. Others are anorexic (no appetite). Walking or taking a ride or any jarring motion aggravates pain. Patient does not want to palpate or to be touched on the abdomen.

DIAGNOSIS: ACUTE APPENDICITIS

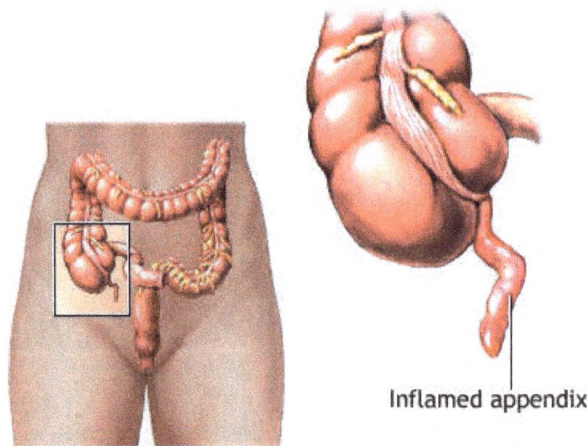

Inflamed appendix

(Show epigastric and hypogastric portion of the abdomen)

ORGAN INVOLVED: *appendix*

CAUSE: *Not known.*

Jogging or any activity could not precipitate the disease. Food is not known to cause it. Familial cause is not a factor.

ADVICE:

No antibiotic could stop the disease. Antispasmodic is not advisable because it could mask the infection in a ruptured appendix. Immediate surgery is advisable to prevent further spread of infection and greater expense. A small incision can be done on the right side of the abdomen if the infection has not spread. Otherwise, a large incision from the epigastric area down to the hypogastrium has to be made to clean the abdomen from pus. If the patient is not operated in due time, the infection spreads throughout the abdomen and the patient may possibly die of SEPTICEMIA (blood poisoning).

LABORATORY EXAMS:

COMPLETE BLOOD COUNT (CBC) – used to determine the presence of infection anywhere in the body though, not specific for acute appendicitis. Any increase of the white blood cells above 10,000 and in the absence of any other focus of infection, such as, in the Upper Respiratory tract is indicative of Acute Appendicitis.

URINALYSIS - to rule out the possibility of *URINARY TRACT INFECTION* that has a similar sign and symptom of Acute Appendicitis.

X- RAY OF THE ABDOMEN - can only indicate that intestine are sides-wept or set aside by pus or in ileus (Intestines are not moving) because of infection. Some may show fecalith or stony feces near the base of the appendix. Thus, it does not help in diagnosis.

ULTRASOUND - does not help in the diagnosis but only rule out the possibility of other diseases like gall bladder stone and kidney stone.

CT SCAN – does not help and even increases expense.

DEFINITIVE TREATMENT:

APPENDECTOMY - an operation performed on the right lower quadrant of the abdomen. A small incision is made at the right side below the navel. This could be horizontal or oblique depending on the surgeon who is doing it. With the appendix right down below the incision, it is pulled up. The base of the appendix is cut and ligated (tied) with an absorbable suture. All pus pooling near the appendix is sucked out and bleeders are also tied. The abdomen is closed layer by layer, (namely) (4 layers: peritoneum, muscles, fatty layer and skin).

EXPLORATORY LAPAROTOMY - an operation done for acute appendicitis which have ruptured or the diagnosis is vague but the symptoms of the patient warrants surgery (Acute Abdomen – term describing an abdominal situation which medical treatment cannot correct and only an operation can save the patient). The incision is made from the top of the abdomen (epigastric) down to the lower portion of the abdomen (hypogastric). All parts of the abdomen are inspected and cleaned (in ruptured Appendicitis) by pouring water inside the abdomen. Appendectomy proper (as described above) is done.

COMPLICATIONS OF SURGERY:

Adhesions – intestines adhere to each other

Bleeding – ties and sutures of the blood vessels loosen.

Pus coming out of the wound – wound becomes infected.

EPIGASTRIC PAIN + LOOSE BOWEL MOVEMENT

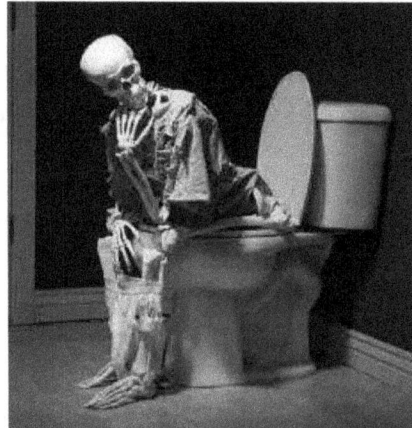

This refers to a pain that starts from the epigastric area and radiates or transfers near the navel associated with loose bowel movement, nausea and vomiting. The pain persists despite defecation and is noted to be colicky and very intense. Stools are noted to be yellowish and scattered like scrambled egg. Abdominal fullness is noted before defecation and persists even after defecation.

DIAGNOSIS: ACUTE GASTROENTERITIS

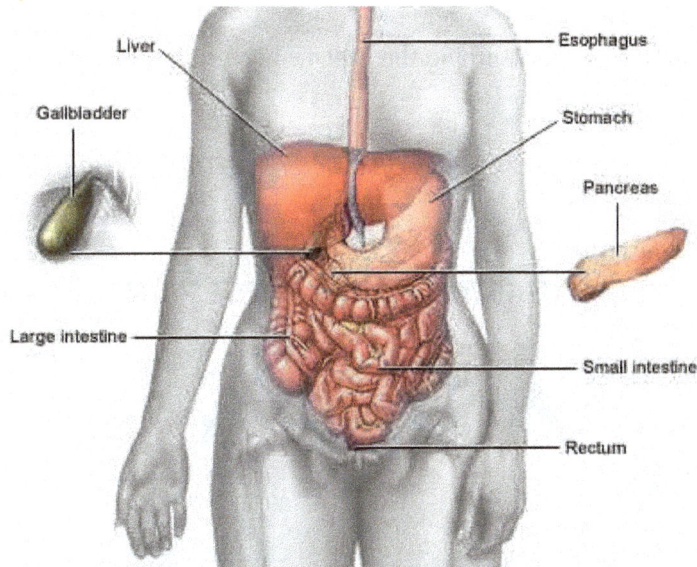

ORGAN INVOLVED: *small intestines*

CAUSE: seasonal, dirty food, unclean food utensils

INITIAL TREATMENT:
> *HYDRATION – lots of water: Hydrite / Glucolyte ORS*
> *BUSCOPAN tablet every 4 hrs. intended for pain.*

ADVICE: Most loose bowel movements end by itself without medications. Proper hydration is the only treatment. But in some cases, (the) bacteria have entered into the food chain and antibiotics are needed for treatment.

LABORATORY EXAMS:

STOOL EXAM – apply to determine the possibility of other cross infections like Amoeba, Typhoid and parasitism, etc.

GRAM STAINS OF STOOLS - to determine the specific bacterium causing the loose bowel movement.

DEFINITIVE TREATMENT:

Adult: OFLOXACIN 200 mg 1 tab 2x 5 days **OR** *children: SEPTRIN SYRUP 1 tsp. 2x a day for 1 week*

EPIGASTRIC PAIN + CHEST PAIN

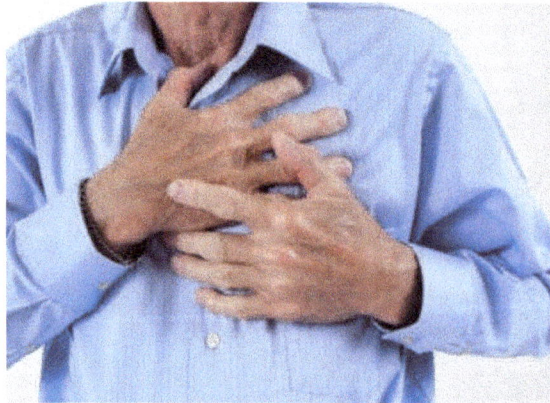

Pain in the epigastrium associated with chest fullness or chest pain is best described as constricting with numbness radiating to the left upper extremity. Sometimes, it occurs in the left jaw with cold sweats and palpitation. This usually leads to loss of consciousness or dizziness.

DIAGNOSIS: medical term: ***myocardial infarction.*** The mild form of chest pains may not be severe and this is called ANGINA.

ORGAN INVOLVED: *heart*

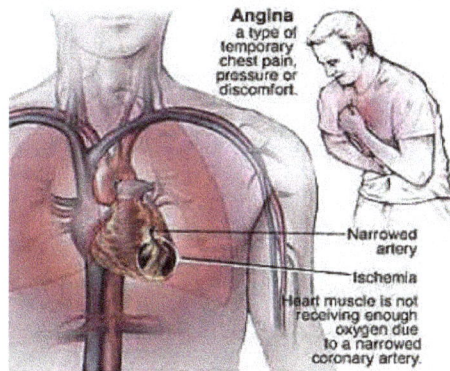

CAUSE:

The arteries of the heart are blocked due to high cholesterol, or embolus.

INITIAL TREATMENT:

Let the patient lie flat. Get towels soaked with warm water and place it on the chest of the patient. If he is taking medications for the heart, let him place one under his tongue. Usually these drugs are in form of NITRITES such as, ISORDIL SUBLINGUAL. Immediate transfer to the hospital is the only way for survival.

ADVICE: A patient should undergo annual blood examination conducted to determine the level of cholesterol, presence of diabetes mellitus; ECG preferably with TREAD MILL could check the impending presence of a heart attack. Lifestyles or moderate exercise, lean food (intake) and (managing) low stress (can reduce) control the incidence of mortality.

LABORATORY EXAMS:

ECG- ELECTROCARDIOGRAM is the fastest way of diagnosing heart attacks. Electrical wirings are attached to the chest connected to a machine, which reads the electrical impulse generated by the heart. Abnormalities of the lines created by the machine indicate diseases like heart attack.

CORONARY ANGIOGRAM is used to determine the location and extent of the blocked blood vessels of the heart. A small tube is inserted thru a vein in the arm or neck and threaded direct into the heart. A dye is injected and an x-ray is done (performed) at the same time.

CT SCAN only determines the extent of the heart damaged by the blockade.

ULTRASOUND (2D ECHOCARDIOGRAM) only used to determine valvular and anatomic cardiac defects.

CHEST X- RAY does not have any role in the diagnosis of heart attack but only determines other damage organs, such as the lungs.

DEFINITIVE TREATMENT:

MEDICATION: *ISOSORBIDE DINITRITE* 1 tab 3 times a day.

CORONARY BYPASS – is a surgical procedure wherein a vein from the thigh of the patient is (removed and) transplanted into the heart to bypass a clogged portion similar to a "flyover" road complex.

CORONARY STENT - a spring-like small contraption is inserted thru a vein in the neck and threaded into the coronaries of the heart to open up the clogged portion of the artery. No major surgical procedure is done but a small wound is made in the neck where the instrument is inserted to carry the "spring" to the heart.

EPIGASTRIC PAIN + RIGHT OR LEFT FLANK PAIN

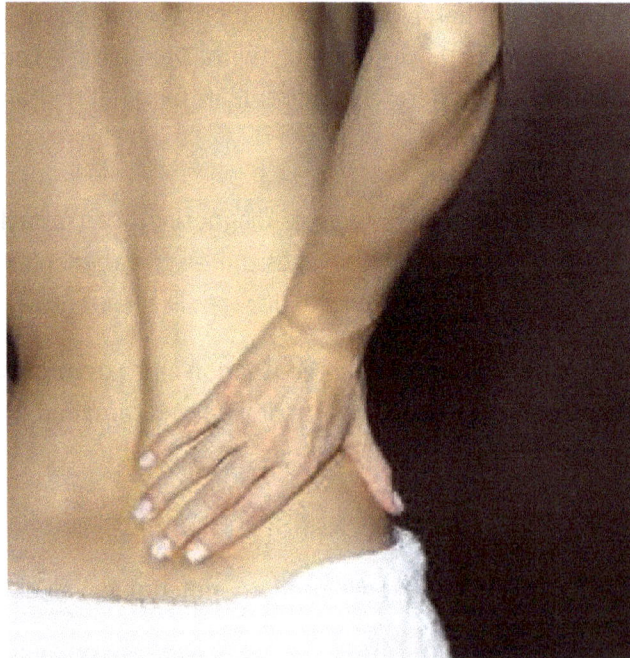

A pain in the epigastrium which radiates to the right or left flank associated with chills and or fever. Sometimes, the pain is noted at the back of the lumbar area. The pain is described to be gnawing or the feeling of heaviness on the side of the abdomen.

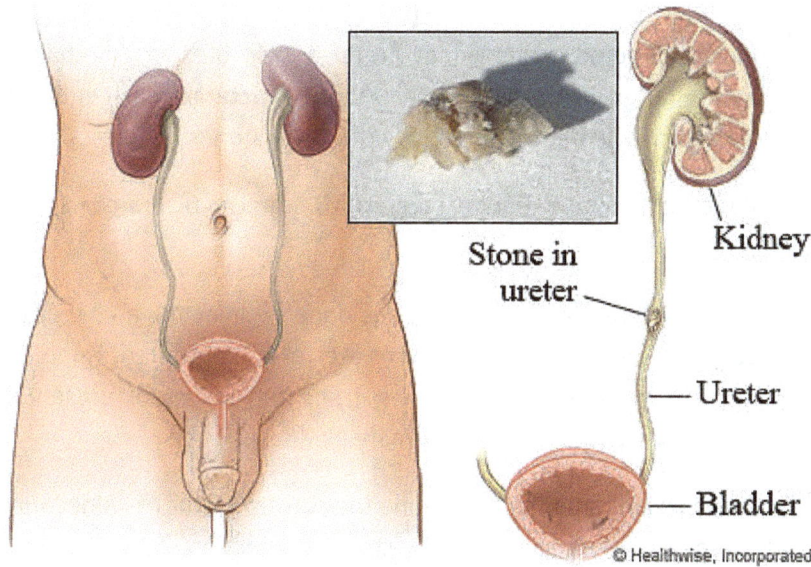

Stone in ureter

Kidney

Ureter

Bladder

© Healthwise, Incorporated

DIAGNOSIS: INFECTION OF THE KIDNEY

ORGAN INVOLVED: kidneys

CAUSE: A long history of urinary tract infection (urinary bladder, urethra, or penile area) not completely treated which ascends into the kidneys.

INITIAL TREATMENT:
> *PARACETAMOL 500 mg 1 tab every 4 hrs. for the fever and chills*
> *BUSCOPAN tablet every 4 hrs. for the abdominal pain Hyoscine butyl bromide*

ADVICE:
Definite treatment should be carried out for 7 days or more, or else infection recurs. Urinalysis should be done before and after the treatment course.

LABORATORY EXAMS:

URINALYSIS - an examination of the urine to determine the cause of the pain since both infection and kidney stones manifest almost the same symptoms. Follow up urinalysis should be done after treatment to determine the complete absence of pus in the urine.

ULTRASOUND - Sound is directed to the kidney-ureter-urinary bladder. The back-fire of this sound will be reflected in a TV like monitor giving the silhouette of these structures which determines the extent of the infection, kidney damage and to rule out the possibility of kidney stones.

CT SCAN – can be done but whatever findings seen by CT scan can be matched by ULTRASOUND at a lesser expense.

INTRAVENOUS PYELOGRAM - an x-ray procedure is done by injecting a chemical (contrast media) into the vein in the arm. Several x-ray views and positions are taken in different minute interval. This will show the size of the kidney, its inside structure, stones inside the kidney, if present, the ureter (tube connecting the kidney to the urinary bladder) and the urinary bladder.

CREATININE – is a blood examination to determine the current status of kidney function. This is very important in determining the extent of damage done by stone or infection. Patient must not eat beginning midnight until the blood is extracted before 9 AM the next day.

DEFINITIVE TREATMENT:

Adult: *GATIFLOXACIN 400 mg 1 tab daily 3 days OR*
CIPROFLOXACIN 500 mg 2x a day for 7 days
Children: *SEPTRIN SYRUP tsp. 2x a day for 1 week*

RIGHT UPPER QUADRANT PAIN

This is a pain felt in the right upper portion of the abdomen, which is aggravated by fatty food intake. The pain is described as piercing often associated with numbness or gnawing pain at the back, bloatedness and the urge to defecate or pass flatus. This is often seen in fat, female, or robust person in the middle ages (35 – 55 yrs.). There is an urge to burp to relieve the pain or to relieve bloatedness.

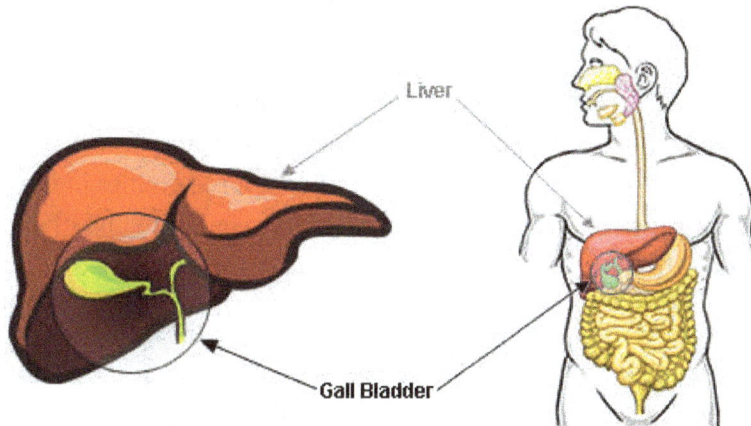

DIAGNOSIS: ACUTE CHOLECYSTITIS – CHOLELITHIASIS

ORGAN INVOLVED: *gall bladder*

CAUSE: infection of the gall bladder or formation of stones in the gall bladder due to high intake of cholesterol rich food.

INITIAL TREATMENT:

> **To dissolve the stone-**ROWACHOL 1 tab 3x day for 3 months pinene 17 mg, camphene 5 mg, cineol 2 mg, menthone 6 mg, menthol 32 mg, borneol 5 mg, olive oil 32 mg
> *High intake of fruits: lemon juice, pineapple, and apple juice*
> **To prevent abdominal pains** - no fatty food in the diet.

ADVICE:

Cholecystitis is infection and swelling of the gall bladder while *Cholelithiasis* is the presence of stones in the gall bladder. Both of these diseases present similar symptoms. If pain is tolerable, surgery can be postponed but the disease may progress due to the enlargement of the stones and/or aggravation of infection. In due course, surgery may become complicated and much more dangerous. In multiple small stones, the danger of dislodging the stones into the common bile duct is very high which may result to obstruction manifested by yellowish discoloration of the eyes.

LABORATORY EXAMS:

ULTRASOUND OF THE GALL BLADDER – is a definitive diagnostic exam that could differentiate the disease from any other forms of abdominal pain. This is done in consonance with ultrasound of the liver, common bile duct, pancreas, and kidneys to determine possible disease entities in these areas, which may present the same symptoms. Patient should not take any food from midnight until the procedure is done at 8am the following day.

CT SCAN – is indicated (resorted to) when entertaining possible malignant disease and/or involvement of other organs nearby like stomach, common bile duct, and pancreas which could not be properly visualized by ultrasound. It is also used to determine the extent of involvement of other organs like cancer when contemplating surgery. The cost prohibits the common use of this diagnostic tool in the diagnosis of gall bladder stone / cholecystitis.

X-RAY - is used to be a diagnostic tool before the advent of the ultrasound. Medicines (contrast media) are given a day prior to the exam to visualize the gall bladder.

DEFINITIVE TREATMENT:

CHOLECYSTECTOMY:

OPEN CHOLECYSTECTOMY – A 3 inch wound below the right rib is made and the gall bladder is removed. Five days to 1 week stay in the hospital is advised. Recovery period would last from 45 days to two months.

LAPAROSCOPIC CHOLECYSTECTOMY – 3 small incisions are made, namely: above the umbilicus, below it and at the side. Operation is done with the use of a laparoscope - a small tube used to visualize the gall bladder inside the abdomen without incising a big wound. Less postoperative pain means fast recovery. This technique cannot be used if the gall bladder is infected, bloated or in the presence of the severe peritonitis (infection of the whole abdomen). Some procedures may be reverted to the open method due to difficulty of the procedure. Thus, additional expense may be (incurred by the patient) added. A 3 to 5 day stay in the hospital is advised. The recovery period would last from 10 to 15 days.

RIGHT UPPER QUADRANT PAIN + YELLOW DISCOLORATION OF THE EYES

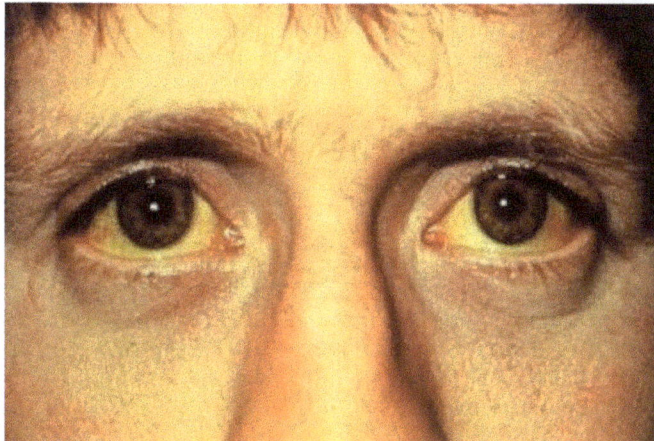

This is best described as apain in the right upper portion of the abdomen accompanied by yellowish discoloration of the eyes; loss of weight, itchiness of the skin, dark color of the urine and grayish color of stools. There is no history of fever in the past two weeks. Mostly found among alcoholics and patients with a history of HEPATITIS B.

DIAGNOSIS: CANCER OF THE LIVER

ORGAN INVOLVED: *liver*

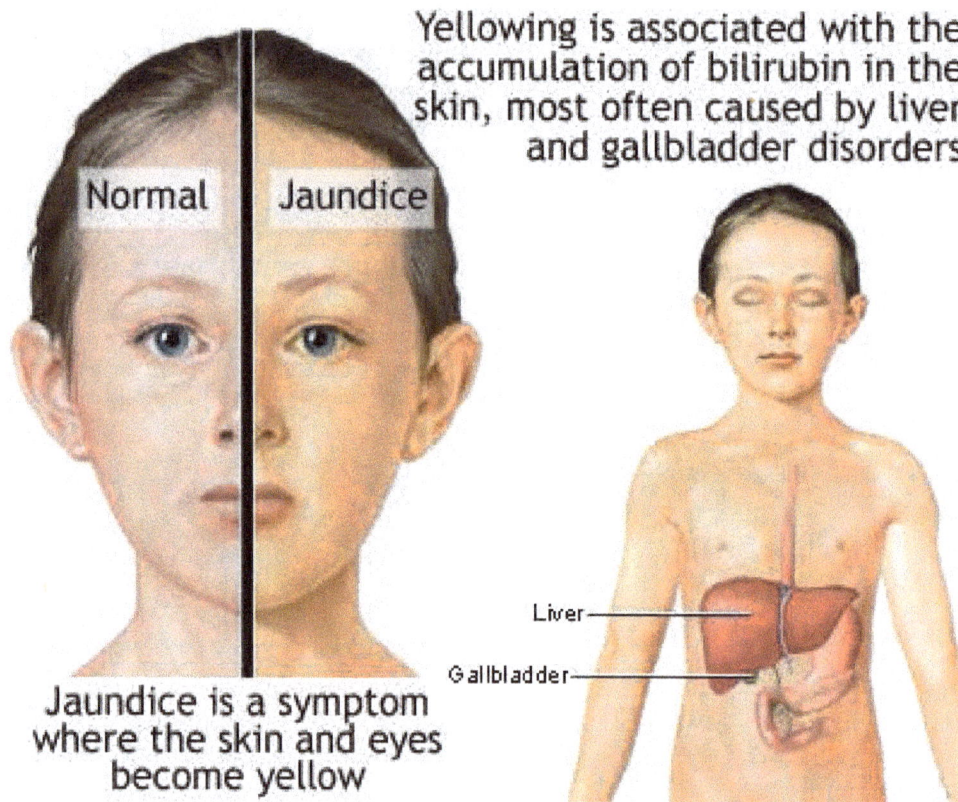

Normal | Jaundice

Jaundice is a symptom where the skin and eyes become yellow

Yellowing is associated with the accumulation of bilirubin in the skin, most often caused by liver and gallbladder disorders

Liver

Gallbladder

CAUSE: not known but there is high association with HEPATITIS B, alcoholism, malnutrition, chemical exposure (pesticide), and drugs.

INITIAL TREATMENT:

For pain – MEFENAMIC ACID 500 mg tablet every 4 hrs. or TRAMADOL 50 mg tablet every 6 hrs.

ADVICE:

Symptoms are vague. Most often, the disease is discovered when it is in the terminal or an incidental finding in a routine checkup. Recent success in the early detection of the disease is done with mass screening of community groups in Japan. Avoidance of food containing aflatoxin, methods of cooking such as smoked fish and BBQ (barbecue cooked meat) and strong food preservatives are not helpful.

LABORATORY EXAMS:

ULTRASOUND – is used as a main detection if there is a tumor in the liver. It is cheap and readily available.

ALPHAFETO PROTEIN – examination of the blood, which confirms the presence of the cancerous tumors in the liver based on the high level of immature protein enzymes.

CT SCAN – it confirms the diagnosis and the extent tumor size, resectability, involvement of other organs.

DEFINITIVE TREATMENT:

LOBECTOMY – surgical removal of a portion of the liver affected by the cancer if it is still localized. If it is affecting the whole liver, liver transplantation is (still) being experimented. Survival rate is 3 to 6 months.

CHEMOTHERAPY – is a less effective method with mean survival rate of 6 – 8 months.

HYPOGASTRIC PAINS + FREQUENCY OF URINATION

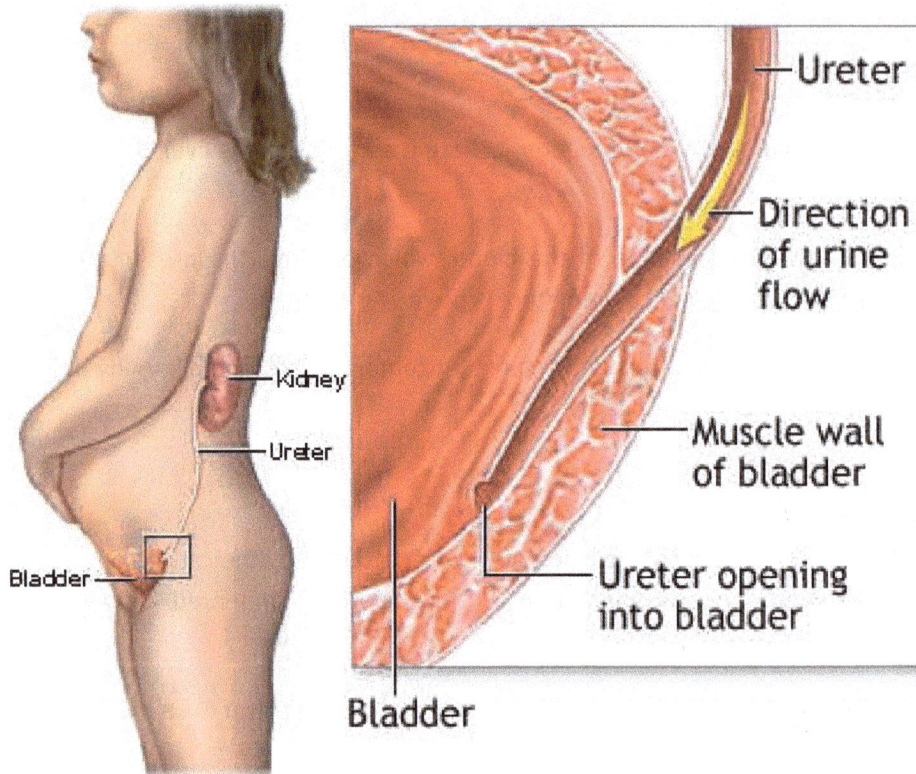

Pains that are located below the abdomen associated with frequent urination, pain during urination, fever, chills.

DIAGNOSIS: URINARY TRACT INFECTION

ORGAN INVOLVED: *urinary bladder*

CAUSE:

Urinary bladder is contaminated due to cross infection, such as: SEXUALLY TRANSMITTED DISEASE, unhygienic practices, presence of stone in the urinary bladder, and retention of urine.

INITIAL TREATMENT:

Frequent and regular vaginal washing in females is recommended. The use of condoms and a regular intake of water are advised.

ADVICE:

Most UTI are caused by sexual transmission whether it is safe or unsafe sex. The proximity of the urethra and anus in the female precludes the extensions of the feces into the vagina. Thus, UTI in females are always recurrent. One (a major) cause of UTI in (among) children is the presence of a long prepuce: one indication of doing circumcision. Definitive treatment should be followed by urinalysis to determine complete eradication of infection.

LABORATORY EXAMS:

URINALYSIS - is the cheapest way to determine infection in the urinary tract.

CULTURE AND SENSITIVITY of urine – to determine the bacteria causing the infection and to determine the specific antibiotic to use.

DEFINITIVE TREATMENT:

TEQUIN 400 mg tablet single dose; GATIFLOXACIN
***Or** INOFLOX 200 mg tablet 2x a day for 5 days; OFLOXACIN*
***Or** CIPROBAY 500 mg tablet 2x a day for 5 days CIPROFLOXACIN*

LEFT LOWER QUADRANT PAIN IN THE ADULT

This is labeled as a pain on the left lower portion of the abdomen accompanied by constipation or intermittent diarrhea and constipation. The feeling of unfulfilled bowel movement or pain before bowel movement is very common. Blood in the stools is often detected and usually followed by relief of the pain. Loss of weight and small caliber of the stool size are some of the signs which could lead to the diagnosis.

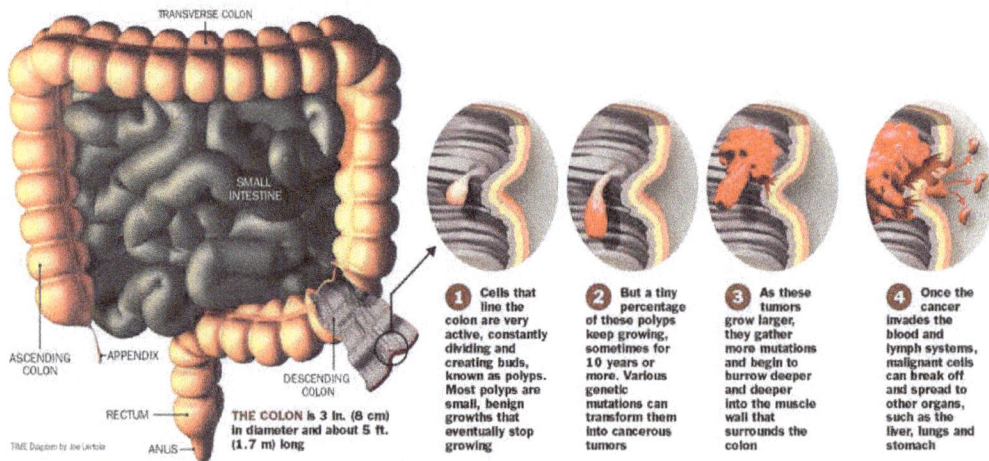

DIAGNOSIS: COLONIC CANCER

ORGAN INVOLVED: *large intestines*

CAUSE: *unknown.*

Chronic cases of Amoebic dysentery, high intake of aflatoxin containing food stuff, high smoke fish and barbecue diet are some of the known factors relating to the incident of colonic cancer.

INITIAL TREATMENT- relieve patient of chronic constipations by means of enema in the form of soapsuds or FLEET ENEMA – a bottled laxative delivered direct to the anus to facilitate bowel movement.

Bisacodyl suppository 1 supp daily; Lactulose; 1 tsp. daily; SENOKOT GRANULES 1 tsp. daily

ADVICE:

Slow progression of symptoms is very common. Most are detected in their late stage. Preventions such as annual physical examination or routine colonoscopy have increased early detection. When found as a partial obstruction, a complete resection without passing through the stage of the colostomy (transfer of stool outlet into the left side of the abdomen) can be done. In late stage, a permanent colostomy after resection is the only option to increase survival.

LABORATORY EXAMINATION:

BARIUM ENEMA – administration of a milk-like substance into the anus prior to taking x-rays of the abdomen. Several films are taken in different angles to locate the tumor.

COLONOSCOPY – using a long fiber-optic tube the size of a ballpen and two arm's length - the whole colon is visualized via a TV monitor.

DEFINITIVE TREATMENT:

HEMICOLECTOMY – is the removal of the involved portion of the large intestines leaving the anus intact for possible reattachment in the near future. Patient has to pass through a colostomy stage wherein the proximal end of the large intestine is brought out through an incision on the left side of the abdomen whereby, the patient moves his feces temporarily via a colostomy bag.

MILES RESECTION – is the complete removal of the lower portion of the large intestine including the anus. This is done in cases where the tumor or cancer is very near the anal area and reattachment of remaining colon to the anus could not be done. The patient permanently moves his bowel through a COLOSTOMY – the proximal portion of the remaining large intestine brought out through a wound on the left side of the abdomen and a bag collects the feces.

LEFT LOWER QUADRANT PAIN IN THE YOUNG

Abdominal pains in children are usually located in the left lower quadrant area associated with constipation, nausea, or vomiting with abdominal bloatedness. When the child is able to defecate, his or her stools are streaked with mucoid blood. A mass is palpable in the left lower quadrant of the abdomen and is tender to touch.

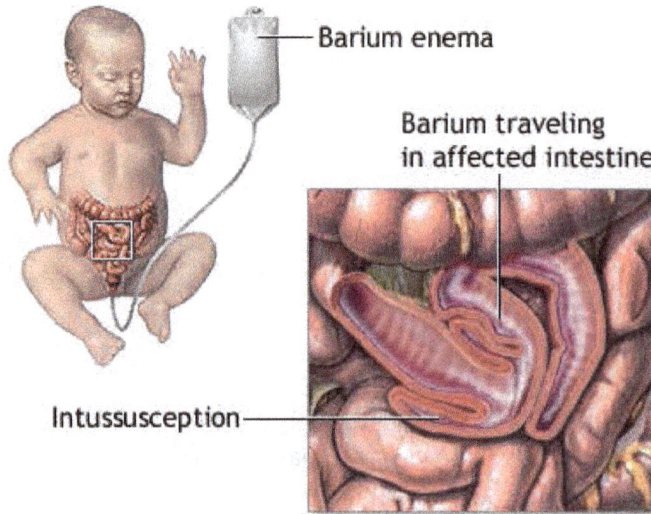

Barium enema

Barium traveling in affected intestine

Intussusception

DIAGNOSIS: INTUSSUSCEPTION

ORGAN INVOLVED: *large intestine*

CAUSE:

A lower portion of the large intestine has inserted itself into the upper portion causing intestinal obstruction.

INITIAL TREATMENT:

The child should not be given any food, made to relax and given an ANTISPASMODIC:
*BENTYL 1 tsp. every 4 hrs.***OR**

*BUSCOPAN Syrup 1 tsp. every 4 hrs.**OR Hyoscine N Butylbromide***
BARALGIN Syrup 1 tsp. every 4 hrs.

LABORATORY EXAMINATION:

UPRIGHT FILM OF THE ABDOMEN – is applied to determine the presence of intestinal obstruction; a scouting film which would show air- fluid level. A pathognomonic sign: COILSIGN would give a probable diagnosis of INTUSSUSCEPTION.

ULTRASOUND OF THE ABDOMEN – cannot help in the diagnosis
CT SCAN – cannot help in the diagnosis either.

ADVICE:

Low pressure barium enema is attempted in children whose cases are early; no fever, no signs of infection in the abdomen, such as, muscle guarding or tenderness on palpation. In most cases, resolution of the illness can be done by mere barium enema. Recurrence may occur and is therefore, an indication to do surgery to look for the possible cause of the INTUSSUSCEPTION.

BARIUM ENEMA – is a diagnostic as well as THERAPEUTIC. Delivery of the low - pressure enema into the anus could free the invaginated intestine.

DEFINITIVE TREATMENT:

EXPLORATORY LAPAROTOMY – a large incision is made on the abdomen from the upper portion down to the lower portion. This is done because the location of the lesion to the intestine cannot be determined prior to surgery. Then, palpation of the large intestine is done to locate possible lesions like, polyps, which initiated the disease. Total excision of the lesion or segmental resection of the intestine is done and reattachment of the remaining portions of the intestine subsequently follows.

WHOLE ABDOMINAL PAIN IN CHILDREN + NO BOWEL MOVEMENT FOR 24 HRS

Abdominal pains in children associated with vomiting, abdominal bloatedness, severe tenderness of the abdomen and no bowel movement for 24 hrs. This is often described as colicky since children suddenly cry but stops abruptly. Some children wreath with pain without let up.

DIAGNOSIS: VOLVULUS

ORGAN INVOVLED: *small intestine*

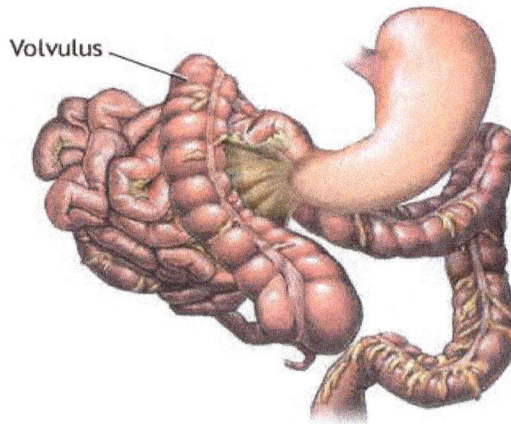

CAUSE: twisting and knotting of the small intestines

INITIAL TREATMENT: *none*
Do not feed the patient even with water.

ADVICE:

Small intestines in children sometimes suddenly knot itself without reason. But in some cases, tumors lead the process or infection initiates the VOLVULUS. The abdominal pain is very severe unlike any other. The child would not stop crying. Medications afford no relief. In examination, the abdomen is so tender that the child would not allow the doctor to touch it. A tube is inserted through her nose upon admission to relieve obstruction.

LABORATORY EXAMINATION:

UPRIGHT FILM OF THE ABDOMEN – an x-ray is taken with the patient standing up or the x-ray table is tilted upwards. This is done to bring down water in the intestine to level off. Presence of water leveling off inside the intestine similar to the steps of a ladder signifies intestinal obstruction.

Ultrasound and CT scan cannot help.

COMPLETE BLOOD COUNT - this examination will show rising infection in the blood as increased number of white blood cells.

DEFINITIVE TREATMENT:

EXPLORATORY LAPAROTOMY - surgery done on a patient whose diagnosis is not definite but the patient's status show that she has ACUTE ABDOMEN - a state of abdomen where no medication could correct the disease, except, surgery. This is based on the findings that the abdomen is showing massive infection such as:

Muscle guarding
Very tender abdomen
Silent intestines
Bloated abdomen

Based on what is found inside, the location where the intestine is knotting is cut and sutured back together.

RESULT OF TREATMENT:

If immediate surgery is done, the success rate is 100%. Selection of antibiotics has a primary role in the treatment. Delayed surgery is the prime cause of death and morbidity.

HYPOGASTRIC PAINS + VAGINAL SPOTTING

This is the pain in the lower portion of the abdomen not accompanying (accompanied with) the usual menstrual period and associated with vaginal spotting usually lasting for several weeks. There is a feeling of hypogastric fullness or enlargement. In some cases, this is mistaken for pregnancy.

DIAGNOSIS: UTERINE MYOMA

ORGAN INVOLVED: *uterus*

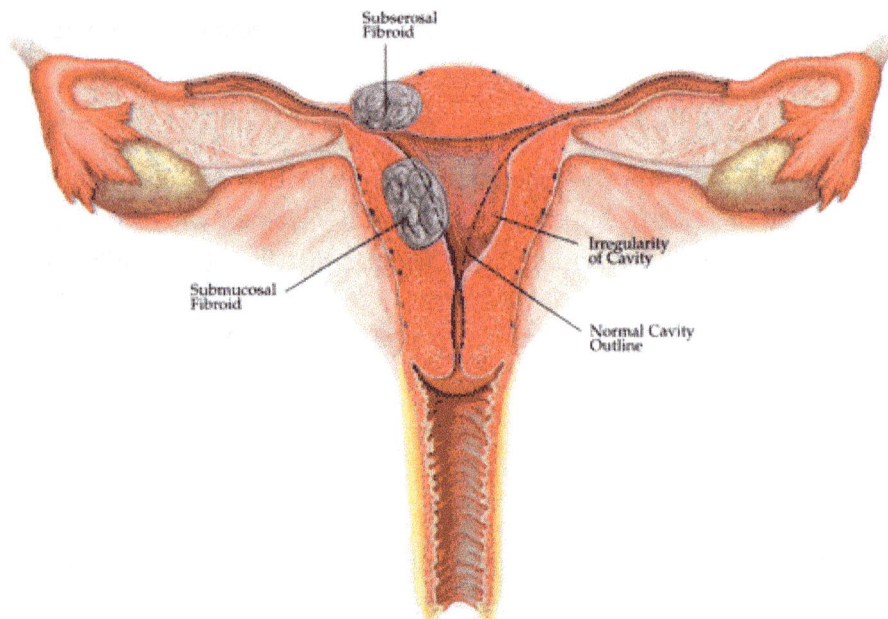

CAUSE: *unknown.*

Some cases have been linked to taking contraceptive pills. Familial history is also linked.

INITIAL TREATMENT:

Alleviation of pain and vaginal bleeding necessitates regular check up with a GYNECOLOGIST.

ADVICE:

Size of the myoma determines the necessity of the surgery and / or the frequency and amount of vaginal bleeding. Childbirth is always taken into consideration.

DEFINITIVE TREATMENT:

HYSTERECTOMY - removal of the uterus which can be done either through the vagina to give a cosmetic effect (VAGINAL HYSTERECTOMY)

ABDOMINAL HYSTERECTOMY – it is done through an open wound on the abdomen.

MYOMECTOMY – enucleation or removal of the myoma inside its shell without removal of the uterus.

HYPOGASTRIC PAINS + MENSTRUATION

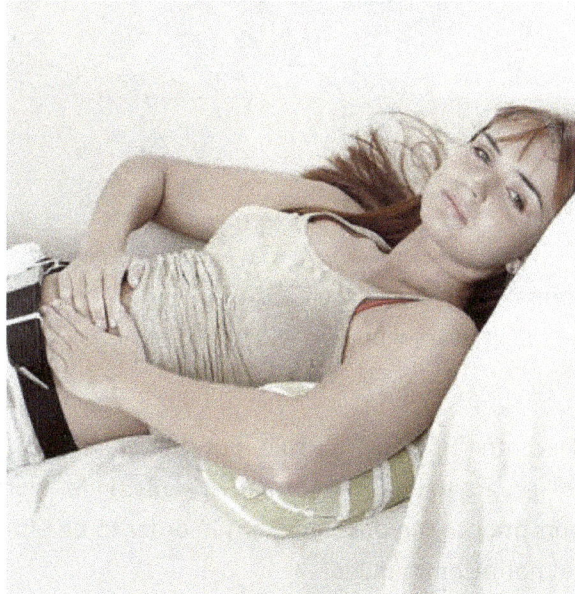

This refers to pains in the lower portion of the abdomen described as crampy in character and usually occurs days before menstruation and during menstruation. Some women may experience body malaise, nausea, dizziness and headache.

DIAGNOSIS: DYSPNEA

ORGAN INVOLVED: uterus

CAUSE:

Due to retroverted uterus, presence of endometriosis (abnormal implantation of inner lining of uterus – endometrium - outside of the uterus); other causes are unknown.

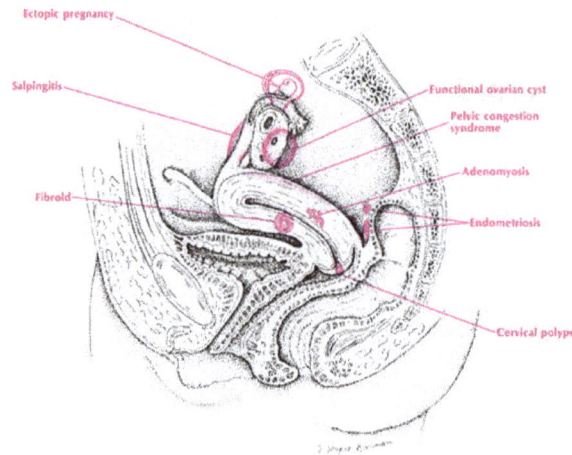

INITIAL TREATMENT: warm compress on the hypogastrium.
MEFENAMIC ACID 500 mg tablet every 4 hours;

ADVICE:

Diagnostic procedures have to be done to rule out the possibility of anatomical or organic abnormality. To take the pains for granted as a normal episode in a woman's cycle is dangerous. Medications have to be taken hours prior to the onset of pains in order to be effective. Massage may help in the cessation of the symptoms but not recommended.

LABORATORY EXAMS:

ULTRASOUND – used to determine the presence of endometriosis or any anatomic abnormality causing the pain during menstruation.

CT SCAN - a very expensive procedure. An Ultrasound can readily detect the (disease and is recommended). It may be used to determine the extent of involvement and respectability (extent of surgery). X- Ray does not help.

DEFINITIVE TREATMENT:

If there is no abnormality found in the diagnostic work up, none is recommended. Presence of endometriosis necessitates removal of the uterus if dysmenorrheal is debilitating.

RIGHT INGUINAL PAIN (OR LEFT) + MASS IN THE SCROTUM

This pain occurs above the inguinal ligament triggered by prolonged standing or walking associated with pain on the right scrotal area and enlargement of the scrotum and / or bulging of the right inguinal ligament area. Lying down and raising the buttocks above the level of the chest relieves pain. Some would be relieved by slowly massaging the mask back into the abdominal area.

DIAGNOSIS: RIGHT INGUINAL HERNIA

ORGAN INVOLVED: abdominal wall defect

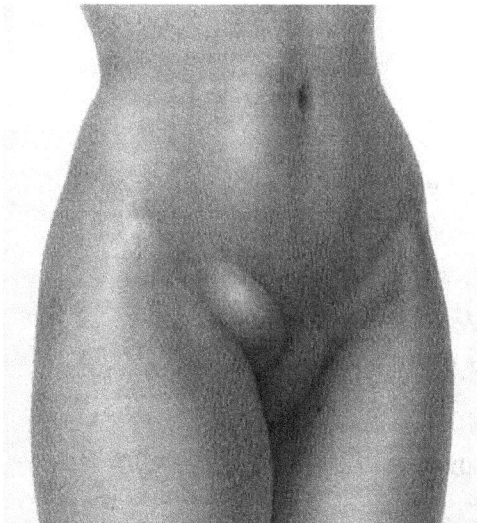

CAUSE:

This is due to a congenital weakness of the abdominal wall and /or failure of the inguinal canal to close at the intrauterine stage in the womb.

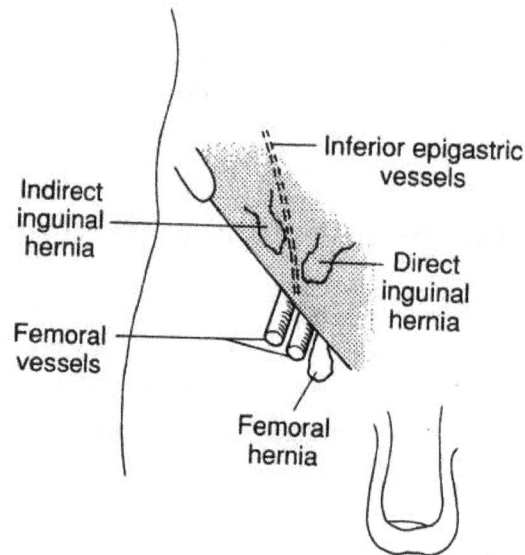

INITIAL TREATMENT:

Use of supporters and constant retraction of the mass back to the abdominal cavity are applied. Refraining from carrying heavy loads may defer surgery **temporarily** but does not cure it.

ADVICE:

This defect is often noted during childhood when the scrotum of the child enlarges during fits of crying. It can also be seen in women but manifest differently with the enlargement of the area above or at the side of the vagina.

LABORATOY EXAMS: None. X-ray does not help either.

DEFINITE TREATMENT:

HERNIORRHAPHY – repair of the abdominal wallet defect by closure of the inguinal canal. 4 -7 days hospital stay. Healing period 45 days to 2 months.

RIGHT OR LEFT FLANK PAIN

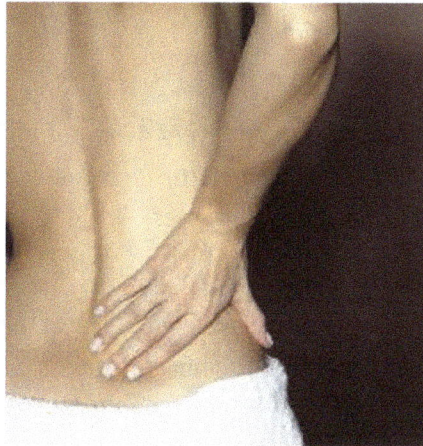

Abdominal pain that is located at the right flank or side of the abdomen radiating to the scrotum or at the side of the thigh. This is also associated with dark colored urine or prank blood in the urine.

DIAGNOSIS: KIDNEY STONE

ORGAN INVOLVED: kidneys – ureter

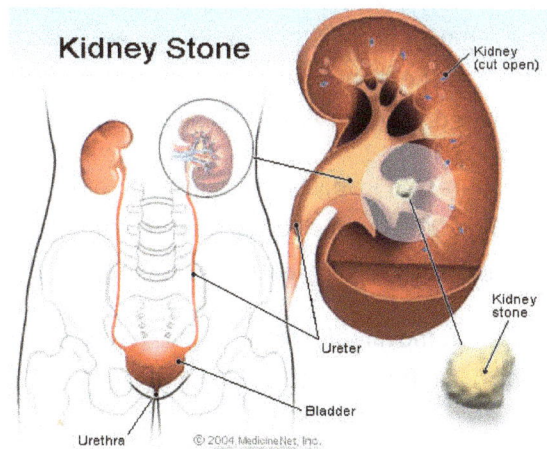

CAUSE:

Formation of hard kidney stone usually made of calcium which sometimes travels down the ureter - tube connecting the kidney down to the urinary bladder.

INITIAL TREATMENT:

BUSCOPAN (Hyoscine N butylbromide) tablet every 4 hrs. for pain. Buko (coconut) juice may help in the dissolving kidney stones. Experiments has been undertaken to know how effective it is.

ROWARINEX tablet 3x a day may dissolve the stones.

ADVICE:

Kidney stones usually form in people who have high uric acid, high purine diet, and high cholesterol blood level. But some people do not have a predetermining factor.

LABORATORY EXAMS:

URINALYSIS – initial exam that could discover the problem by the presence of blood in the urine.

ULTRASOUND – it is accurate, cheap and readily available.

INTRAVENOUS PYELOGRAM – pinpoints location of the stone by x-ray but involves injection of contrast media, which may trigger allergy.

DEFINITIVE TREATMENT:

PYELOLITHOTOMY - is the removal of the stone in the kidney. A large wound is made on the side of the patient extending from the back to the front. The kidney is split open and the stone is removed in toto. 10-15 days stay in the hospital is advised. Recovery period would last from 2 to 4 months.

LITHOTRIPSY – a non-surgical procedure and involves bombardment of kidney stone by ultrasonic device. Its cost ranges from P120, 000 to P130, 000. A repeat of procedure may have to be done to dissolve stones. Failure cases are common. Side effects such as liver laceration and organ hematoma occur.

URETEROLITHOTOMY – the removal of stone in the ureter. A stay of 4 -7 days hospital is recommended. Healing period would last from 10 -15 days.

SCROTAL PAINS

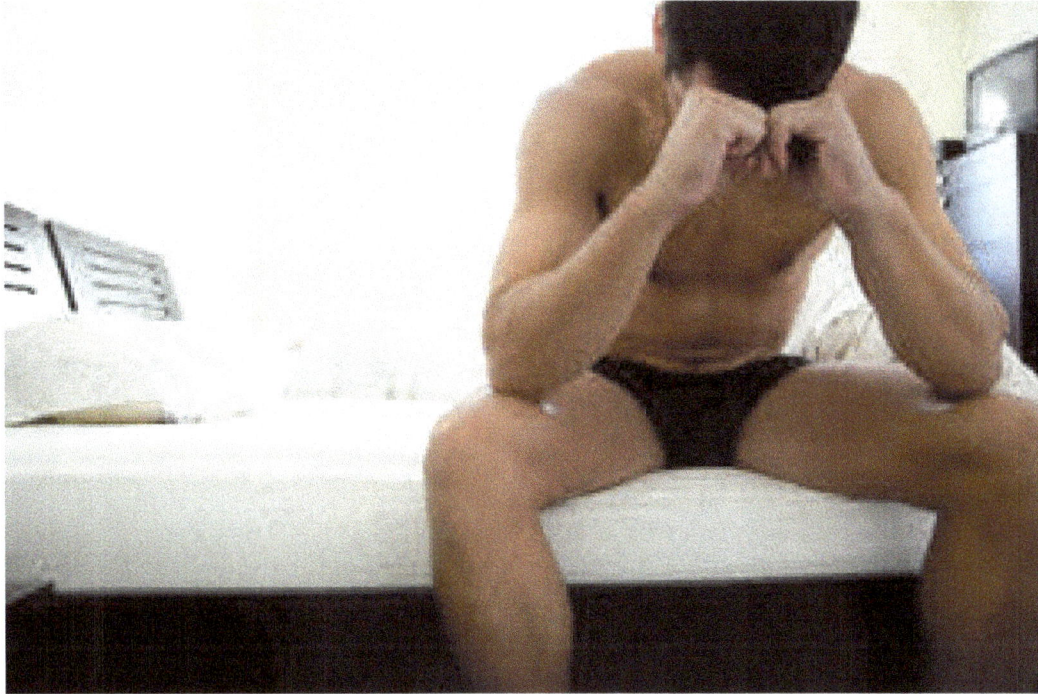

Pains in the scrotum are common in young male adults. These are often due to infections and most commonly caused by sexually transmitted disease.

Male Reproductive Tract

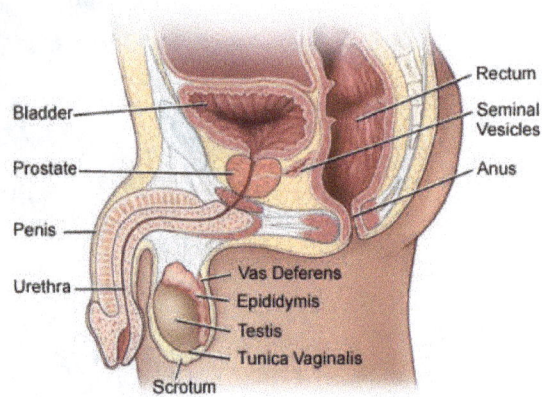

A history of urinary tract infection with incomplete treatment precedes the pain. The testicle is very tender and any jarring movement aggravates the pain. This is associated with swelling of the whole testicle. However, there are other diseases that may cause this pain. Follow the schema below to find the diagnosis and the treatment.

PAIN IN THE SCROTUM IN MUMPS

Some patients develop pain in the scrotum after a high grade fever associated with mumps. Though, not all patients develop this complication, if found in males, it may lead to sterility.

DIAGNOSIS: MUMPS ORCHITIS

CAUSE: invasion of the mumps virus into the testicles

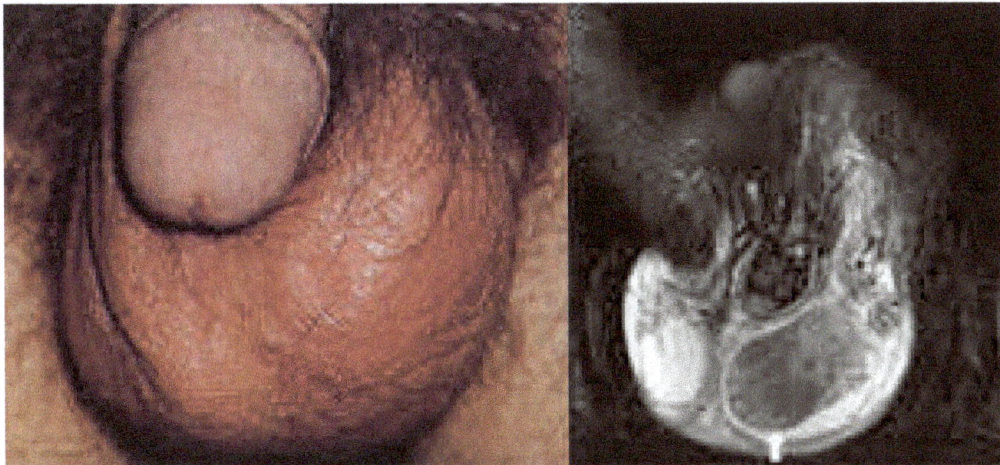

INITIAL TREATMENT:

MEFENAMIC ACID 500 mg tablet every 4 hrs. for pain

LABORATORY EXAMINATION:

ULTRASOUND OF THE SCROTUM – This is done to rule out the possibility of other illnesses, which may manifest as pain in the scrotum. Otherwise, no definitive finding is found in cases like this.

URINALYSIS - to determine the presence of bacteria in the urine which may have triggered the cross infection into the testicles.

DEFINITIVE TREATMENT:

VALTREX 500 mg tablet 3x a day for 10 days. Clinical trials are still going on whether this drug could help in the treatment of MUMPS orchitis.

Swelling of the tube at the side of the testicle collects and stores the sperm before ejaculation.

This often follows an episode of urinary tract infection due to sexually transmitted disease or infection of E. coli. A tender longitudinal mass is palpable on the side of the scrotum. The testis is noted to be soft and non – tender.

DIAGNOSIS: ACUTE EPIDIDYMITIS

CAUSE: infection of the epididymis

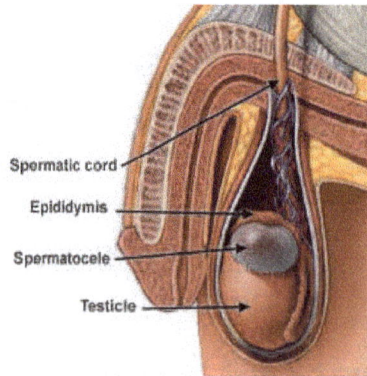

INITIAL TREATMENT:

MEFENAMIC ACID 500 mg 1 tab every 4 hrs

ADVICE:

Incomplete treatment of ordinary urinary tract infection leads to the infection of the epididymis. Thus, a follow- up urinalysis should be done after treatment of UTI to determine the persistence of bacteria in the urine. Antibiotics have difficulty in entering the area of scrotum. Specific antibiotics are recommended. Frequent ejaculation hastens the decrease of swelling.

LABORATORY EXAMINATION:

URETHRAL SMEAR - With the use of a glass slide, a smear of the penile discharge is examined. Identification of the bacteria thru this method determines the specific antibiotic to use.

URINALYSIS - determines the presence of UTI.

DEFINITIVE TREATMENT:

Gatifloxacin 400 mg 1 tab daily for 5 days

PAIN IN THE SCROTUM IN VARICOCELE

This refers to the convolution of the blood vessels, mostly the veins of the scrotum draining the testes causing swelling and pain on the side of the scrotum.

CAUSE: Unknown. Men who carry heavy weights have predilection or are prone to this type of disease.

INITIAL TREATMENT:

For pain- *Mefenamic 500 mg tablet every 4 hrs* ***OR***
Diclofenac Na 50 mg tablet every 4 hrs

ADVICE:

Straining in carrying heavy load predisposes men to this disease. But other men develop this illness even without the predisposing factor. Some people may live with it without treatment. But others develop sterility / impotence due to this disease. A palpable long mass is noted on the side of the scrota, above the testis, which feels like a hard string with convolutions on some parts. Diagnosis depends on the physical examination.

LABORATORY EXAMINATION:

ULTRASOUND OF THE SCROTUM - Some sonologists could visualize the problem. But others may have difficulty.

PAIN IN THE SCROTUM IN TESTICULAR TORSION

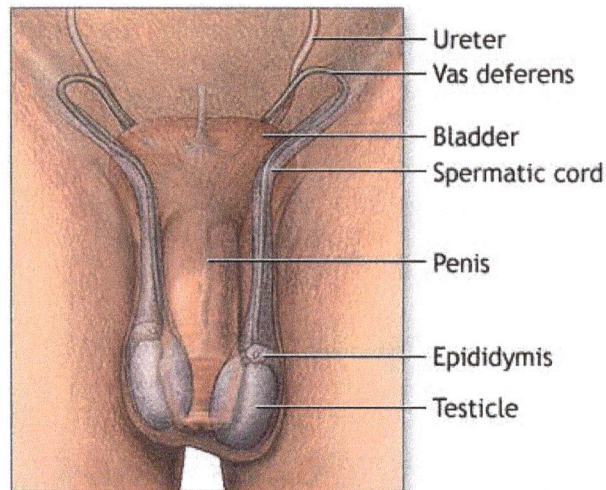

The irrational turning of the testis on its own axis causing torsion of the vas deferens and blood vessels found in the pedicle of the scrotum.

CAUSE: Unknown. Straining in carrying heavy load may cause it.

INITIAL TREATMENT:
MEFENAMIC ACID 500 mg tablet every 4 hrs for pain

ADVICE:
Immediate surgery is the only choice of treatment. Delay in the treatment may cause severe swelling of the testicles followed by necrosis and destruction of the testes involved.

DEFINITIVE TREATMENT:
SURGERY – detorsion and salvaging of the testis if still viable. Otherwise, removal of the testis involved is necessary to prevent infection.

PAINS OF THE CHEST AND BREAST PAINS

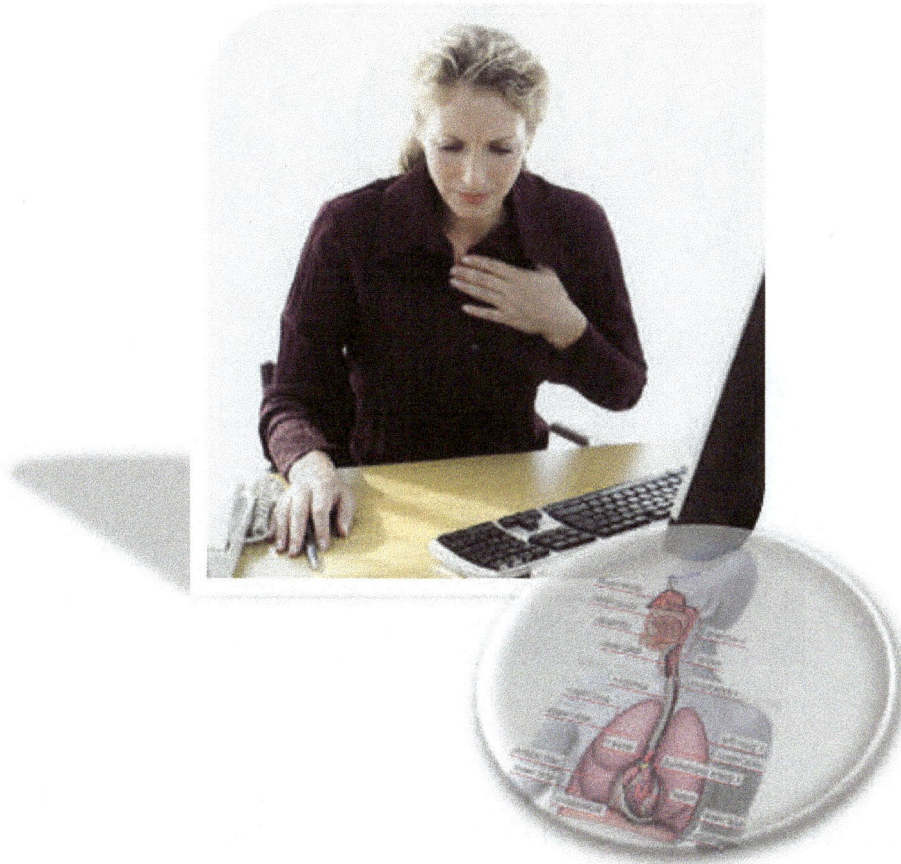

Pains in the chest are most commonly due to two organs: HEART AND LUNGS, which dominate the content of the CHEST cavity. The other organ, which could be the source of pain, is the esophagus, found at the upper portion of the stomach, diaphragm, the great blood vessels, breast in women and the bones making the chest itself. Unlike the abdomen, pains in the chest are mostly associated with difficulty of breathing, shortness of breath, and marked exhaustion.

CHEST PAIN + NUMBNESS OF LEFT ARM

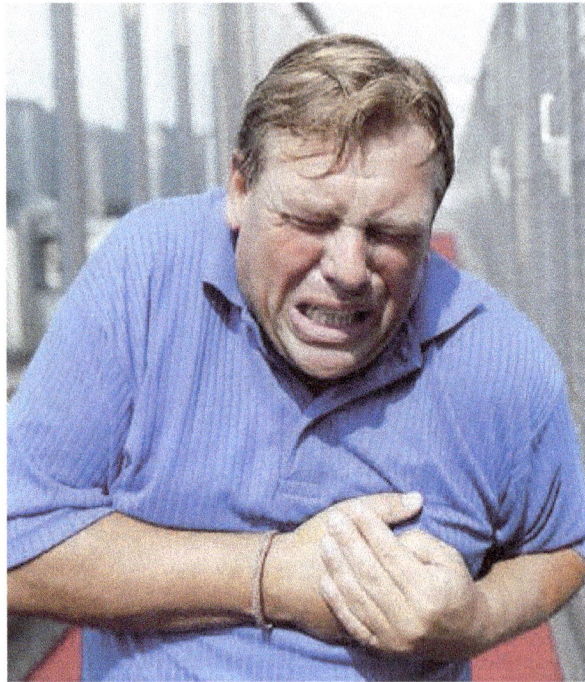

Chest pains constricting or stabbing in character located below the left nipple associated with numbness of the left arm and / or numbness of the lower jaw. This is followed by dizziness, difficulty of breathing, pallor and profuse cold sweats.

DIAGNOSIS: HEART ATTACK

ORGAN INVOLVED: *heart*

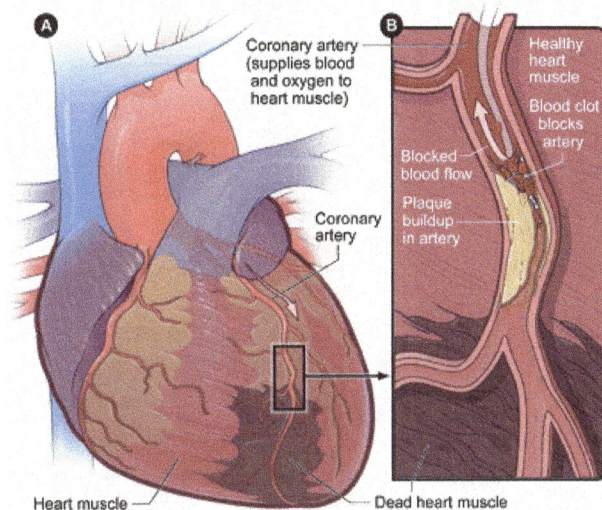

Coronary artery (supplies blood and oxygen to heart muscle)

Healthy heart muscle

Blood clot blocks artery

Blocked blood flow

Plaque buildup in artery

Coronary artery

Heart muscle

Dead heart muscle

INITIAL TREATMENT:

Let the patient lie down comfortably with a pillow. Apply warm compress on the chest on top of the heart or any liniment that could bring heat to the painful area of the chest. If patient has its own medicine with him, place a tablet (ISORDIL SUBLINGUAL) under his tongue. If ever, ask him or her to drink warm water, not cold (to bring blood circulation into his chest).

BRING HIM IMMEDIATELY TO THE HOSPITAL.

Survival is high when patient is brought to the hospital in 5 minutes. The fastest that an ambulance could reach you is 15 minutes. Bringing the patient to the hospital yourself is the best decision.

ADVICE:

Stress or any intense physical activity may precipitate the attack most likely in people above 30 years old, obese and hypertensive. Most attacks come suddenly but others may have pre-attack symptoms like palpitation, dizziness, weakness, and drowsiness.

DEFINITIVE TREATMENT:

See *EPIGASTRIC PAINS + CHEST PAINS*

CHEST PAINS + HYPERACIDITY

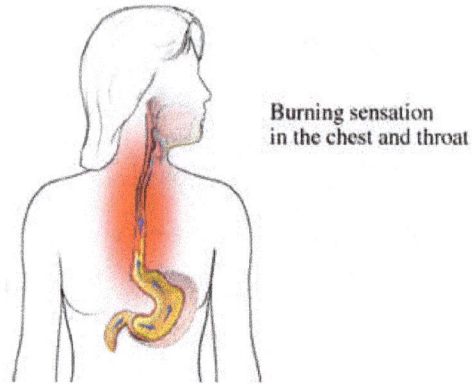

Burning sensation
in the chest and throat

Chest pains located on the center of the chest, which seemed to radiate all over associated with hyperacidity, abdominal fullness and sometimes back pains.

DIAGNOSIS: REFLUX ESOPHAGUS – HEARTBURN

ORGAN INVOLVED: *esophagus*

CAUSE:

Hyperacidity of the stomach which backfires to the esophagus due to the weakness of the esophageal sphincter located above the stomach causing retrograde flow of acid. Some of the possible causes are the following: overeating, obesity, reclining immediately after eating and stress.

INITIAL TREATMENT:

ANTACIDS – KREMIL – S 1 tab every 2 hrs. until relief **OR**
MAALOX 1 tab every 2 hrs. **OR** *Aluminum / Magnesium antacid*
NOVALUCID 1 sachet every 2 hrs.

ADVICE:

Most patients who suffer with reflux esophagitis have a running bout of HYPERACIDITY, PEPTIC ULCER, or both. Refraining from reclining or lying down immediately after meals, overeating and acidic foods prevents pain.

DEFINITIVE TREATMENT:

Repair of the esophageal sphincter which necessitates surgery across the chest or approached thru the abdomen. Within10 - 15 DAYS HOSPITAL STAY is highly recommended. 30 days recovery period is needed.

CHEST PAIN + PAIN ON INSPIRATION

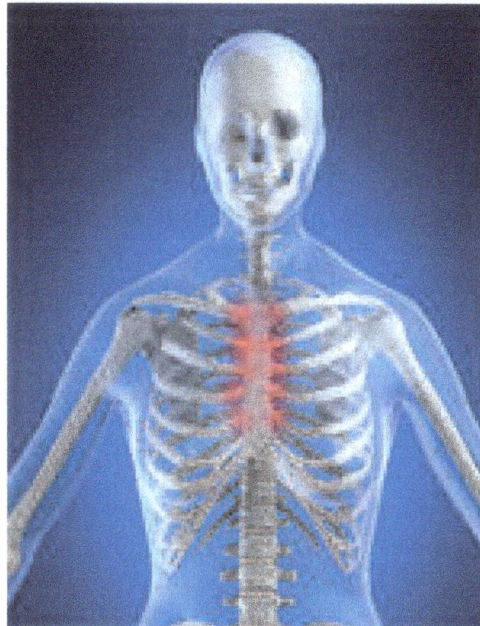

Pain on the chest radiates to the left side near the heart. No cold sweats palpitation and dizziness. It is aggravated by moving or extending the upper extremity and taking a deep breath. Pain is usually noted at the right side of the sternum.

DIAGNOSIS*:* COSTOCHONDRITIS

ORGAN INVOLVED: *ribs and sternum*

CAUSE:

  Arthritis is the swelling of the costochondral junction of the ribs, the junction between the cartilaginous and bony portion of the chest. History of trauma is often noted.

INITIAL TREATMENT:

  IBUPROFEN tablet every 4 hrs. **OR**
  MEFENAMIC tablet every 4 hrs. **OR**
  (DICLOFENAC NA 50 mg tablet every 6 hrs.) / MELIXICAM 15 mg tablet daily

ADVICE:

  No amount of massage could alleviate pain. Rest and proper diet could prevent further episodes of pain. Medications have to be taken for more than 2 weeks to prevent reoccurrence.

LABORATORY EXAMINATION:

  ECG – used to rule out the possibility of an impending heart attack.

  X-ray of the THORACIC BONY CAGE - to determine the magnitude of swelling or the presence of it; fractures could also be detected.

  BLOOD URIC ACID DETERMINATION – used to determine the level of uric acid which is the common cause of gouty arthritis.

DEFINITIVE TREATMENT:

  ETORICOXIB *ARCOXIA 120 mg tablet daily* **OR**
  CELECOXIB (CELEBREX) 200 1cap daily **AND**
  ALLOPURINOL 300 1 tab daily (for those who have a high level of uric acid)

CHEST PAIN + COUGH

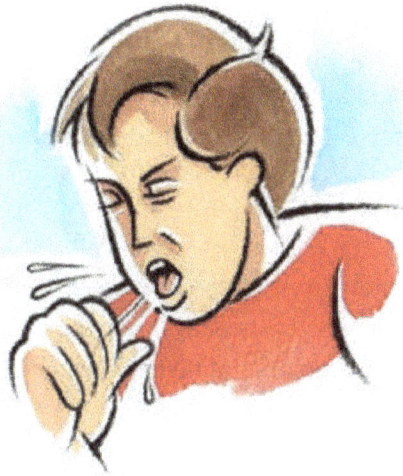

Pain that is located in the lateral side of the chest but sometimes involving the back and front associated with cough and difficulty of breathing.

DIAGNOSIS: PLEURAL EFFUSION

ORGAN INVOLVED: *lungs*

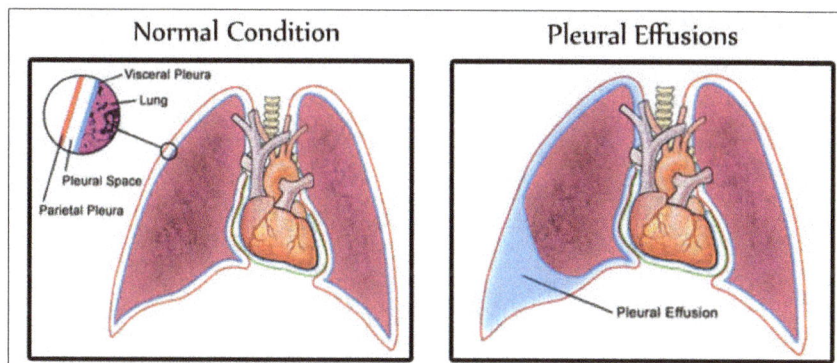

INITIAL TREATMENT: *none*

ADVICE:

Pleural effusion is due to the accumulation of fluid in the lungs secondary to other illness like lobar pneumonia, asthma, congestive heart failure, renal failure, cancer metastasis, allergic reaction and side effects of medications in chemotherapy. Treatment consists of extraction of the fluid in the lungs and the treatment of the main problem.

LABORATORY EXAMINATION:

CHEST X- RAY - fluid is shown on x-ray whitening of otherwise black area in an aerated lung. When small in amount, it usually pools on the side of the lungs near the diaphragm and is described as BLUNTING OF THE COSTOPHRENIC ANGLE. When the amount of fluid is substantial, a wide part of the lateral side of the lungs is covered by a whitish area on x-ray film.

DEFINITIVE TREATMENT:

ANTIBIOTICS - used if the pleural effusion is due to bacterial infection and the amount is minimal.

ANTI – TB DRUGS - used if the pleural effusion is due to tuberculosis. MYRIN –P FORTE 3x a day

THORACENTESIS – the insertion of a long needle into the lungs via the 5th- 7th rib space at the back and aspiration of the fluid by a large syringe.

CHEST TUBE INSERTION - surgical opening of a wound in the space between ribs and insertion of a large tube to drain the fluid into the water sealed bottle – a simple bottle containing water, which prevents air from entering while catching the drainage from the chest.

CHEST PAIN + VESICLE FORMATION

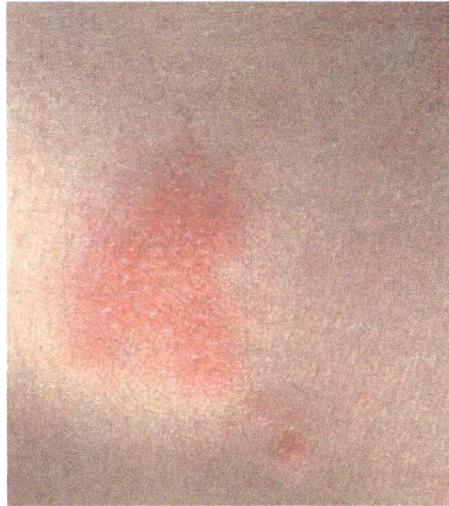

Pain on the side of the chest associated with vesicle formations following the contour of the rib.

DIAGNOSIS: HERPES ZOSTER

ORGAN INVOLVED: *skin*

INITIAL TREATMENT:

> ***For pain*** – *MEFENAMIC ACID 500 mg tablet every 4 hrs.* **OR**
> *TRAMADOL 50 mg tablet every 6 hrs.* **OR** *Tramadol hydrocloride*
> *BEXTRA 40 mg tablet every 24 hrs. (Veldecoxib)*

ADVICE: This is a viral infection involving the skin and no amount of antibiotics helps. However, liniments may relieve the pain.

DEFINITIVE TREATMENT:

> VALACYCLOVIR 500 mg 1 tab 3x a day for 10 – 15 days

BREAST PAIN IN 18 YR OLD

Pain in the breast of an 18 yr. old usually occurs due to the expansion of the size of the breast due to gradual stimulation of the hormones ESTROGEN. This usually starts at the age of 15 until adulthood and/or pregnancy occurs. No masses are noted.

DIAGNOSIS: NORMAL BREAST EXPANSION

CAUSE: ESTROGEN stimulation of the breast tissue, a normal occurrence in young females.

INITIAL TREATMENT:

ANALGESICS: PARACETAMOL 500 mg tablet every 4 hrs. **OR**
MEFENAMIC 500 mg tablet every 4 hrs. **OR**
IBUPROFEN 50 mg tablet every 6 hrs.

ADVICE:

Most girls in their puberty stage have enlargement of their breasts. This constitutes the pain that they feel usually before, during and after menstruation. Firm bras but not so tight may alleviate the pain. Movement or jarring motions may aggravate the pain. Most masses palpated during this age are indurations or islands of breast tissues which have not expanded. They are not cyst or tumors and do not need surgery or biopsy. Girls whose mothers have large breasts suffer pain most often. Consultation with a general surgeon is a must to determine the presence of tumors or cyst formation.

LABORATORY EXAMINATION:

MAMMOGRAPHY – is not necessary. Exposure to the radiation is a high risk with less benefit at this age.

BREAST SONOGRAM – may be of use to determine the presence of masses that contain liquid. Less likely produce radiation exposure. False negative is greater. False positive is more likely.

DEFINITIVE TREATMENT: Conservative. Further examination has to be done yearly up to the time of pregnancy.

BREAST PAIN IN 25 YR OLD SINGLE

Pain in the breast usually triggered by overwork or physical activity is not associated with nipple discharge or masses.

CAUSE: Most often seen in women who are physically active and have moderately large breasts.

DIAGNOSIS: NORMAL

INITIAL TREATMENT: ANALGESICS as above

ADVICE: It has to be seen by a general surgeon to determine the presence of breast masses. The best time for medical checkup is after menstruation to negate breast engorgement due to estrogen stimulation.

LABORATORY EXAMINATION:

MAMMOGRAPHY - is done in women whose family history is positive for CANCER (mother, aunt, grandparents)

BREAST SONOGRAM – applies for women whose family history is negative for breast cancer.

DEFINITIVE TREATMENT: None if masses are discovered.

BREAST PAIN DURING LACTATION

Pain in the breast during lactation is associated with swelling and tenderness near the nipple or beside it.

DIAGNOSIS: ACUTE MASTITIS

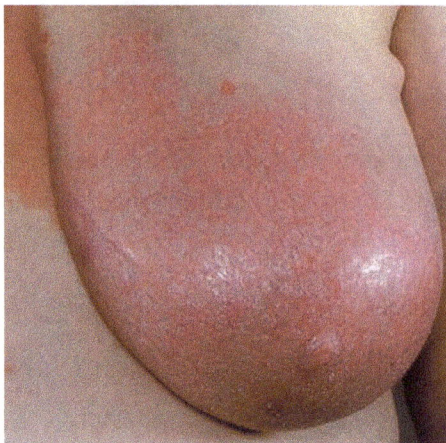

INITIAL TREATMENT:

WARM COMPRESS on the affected area. Wash with soap and water.
MEFENAMIC 500 mg 1 cap every 4 hrs. OR
DICLOFENAC NA 50 mg tablet every 4 hrs.

ADVICE:

This is a bacterial infection due to minute abrasion of the nipple during breastfeeding that allowed entry of bacteria into a rich medium of milk. Prevention can be done by frequent washing of nipple and stoppage of breastfeeding when the nipple gets sore or transferring feeding to the other breast.

DEFINITIVE TREATMENT:

CLOXACILLIN 500 mg 1 cap 4x a day for 7days. If pus formation occurs, an INCISION AND DRAINAGE have to be done to drain out the pus.

BREAST PAIN DURING MENOPAUSE

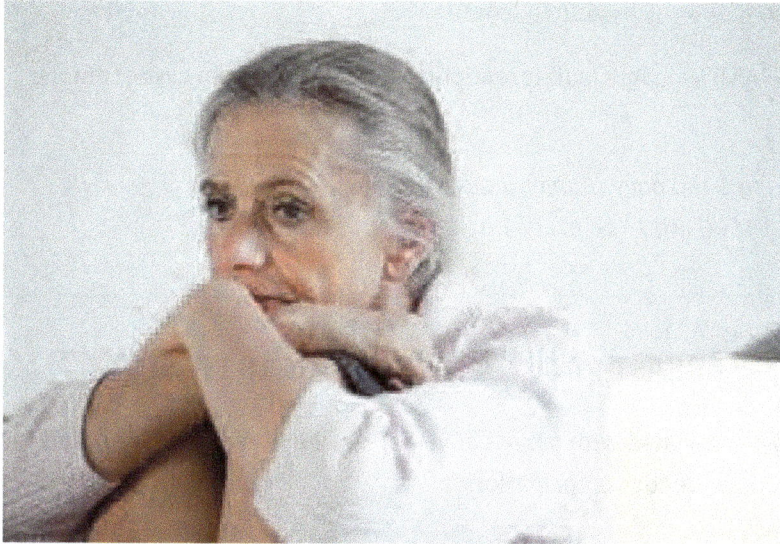

Pain of the breast occurring after the cessation of menstruation usually felt at the early stage and often associated with symptoms of MENOPAUSAL SYNDROME such as flushing irritability, dryness of the skin and vagina and absence of menstruation.

DIAGNOSIS: HYPOGONADISM

INITIAL TREATMENT: Warm compress may help and the use of tight bras during mobility.

ADVICE:

The female breasts are dependent on the estrogen secretion of the ovary such that, in menopause, the absence of estrogen depresses the normal architecture of the breast. Shrinkage of the breast tissues impinges on the pain receptors found in the breast. But other diseases such as malignancy have to be ruled out. Therefore, consultation has to be done with a surgeon to determine the presence or absence of tumors in the breast.

LABORATORY EXAMINATION:

MAMMOGRAPHY: Has to be done if no masses are palpable in the breast to screen out the possibility of non - palpable tumors (less than 5 mm)

BREAST SONOGRAM: Valuable in differentiating solid tumors from cystic tumors.

DEFINITIVE TREATMENT:

PREMARIN 625 mg 1 tab daily (Conjugated estrogens)
MEFENAMIC ACID 500 mg 1 tab every 4 hrs.

BREAST PAIN + A MASS IN AN 18 YR OLD

Pain in the breast associated with a mass anywhere in the breast. Mass is noted to be irregular in shape and sometimes tender on palpation.

DIAGNOSIS: BREAST INDURATIONS, NON – MALIGNANT

CAUSE: Normal breast growth

ADVICE:

Most breast masses in young women are non- malignant and due to unexpended breast tissues. Islands of breast sections do not follow the normal expansion of the rest of the breast thereby, producing pockets of hard masses vague in shape and could not be delineable as significant tumors. These do not require further work up but mere checkup down to the age of 30 years until they reach the age of lactation. By that time, these masses disappear due to milk formation. If this persists after lactation, biopsy then is required.

LABORATORY EXAMINATION: *None.*

Breast sonograms and mammography do not help in discerning the presence of malignancy or benign tumor.

BREAST PAIN + ROUND MASS IN A 21 YR OLD

Pain in the breast associated with rounded mass which moves on palpation and most often very shallow in depth.

DIAGNOSIS: FIBROCYSTIC DISEASE OF THE BREAST

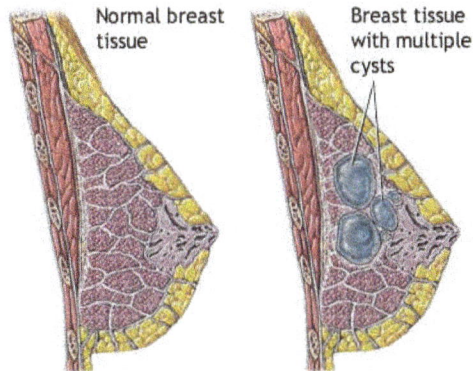

CAUSE: Unknown

INITIAL TREATMENT: None

LABORATORY EXAM:

MAMMOGRAPHY - is only done when no masses are palpable. When a mass is palpable, the procedure is moot and academic.

ADVICE:

These breast masses are noted to grow fast and most often associated with breast pains occurring before, during or after menstruation. Fears of malignancy most often drive the patient or parents to seek medical help. But 95% of these masses are benign and do not require further treatment. The problem lies in the delineation of the malignant from the benign tumors. Thus, a biopsy has to be done in order to identify the mass.

DEFINITIVE TREATMENT:

EXCISIONAL BIOPSY – the whole mass is removed under local anesthesia. Most often, it is done in the clinic. The mass is sent out directly to the laboratory. This medical procedure is preferred by the author in order to remove the anxiety of knowing that some of the tumor still exist inside and there is a possibility of transforming into a malignant form. No section of the mass is left out for definitive diagnosis.

FINE NEEDLE BIOPSY – a large bore of needle is inserted / guided into the mass and a portion of the mass is aspirated with the use of high-pressure syringe. The specimen is then sent to the laboratory for HISTOPATHOLOGIC DIAGNOSIS. If the result is benign, no further treatment is done. However, some surgeons do a second procedure in order to remove the tumor upon the insistence of the patient or the relative.

BREAST PAIN + MASS IN A 35 YR OLD

Pain occurring in the breast associated with a palpable mass.

DIAGNOSIS: RULE OUT MALIGNANCY

INITIAL TREATMENT: None

ADVICE:

Foremost, the mass has to be definitely diagnosed whether it is malignant or not. The high incidence of breast cancer in this age group is alarming. The presence of cancer in the family like mothers, aunts, grandparents should alert the patient to seek medical help. There are several modes on how to do this.

LABORATORY EXAMINATIONS:

FROZEN SECTION – the breast mass is removed under general anesthesia and immediately sent to the laboratory to determine the presence of malignancy with the intention of doing definitive treatment of breast malignancy set-up (removal of the entire breast). The advantage of this set- up is that diagnosis is immediately known; anxiety is minimized; and it's cheaper. The disadvantage of this technique is that the patient is asleep and cannot be informed of the procedure.

FINE NEEDLE BIOPSY – A large bore needle is used to extract a piece of the breast mass and send (sent) to the laboratory for a diagnosis. This can be done in clinic setting; (and the) expense is very minimal. The result is usually available in 7 to 10 days. A second procedure has to be done in order to remove the mass if it is found to be benign. But this technique is more advantageous, in that, the patient can be psychologically prepared before the definitive treatment of removing the entire breast. False negative is high due to the inability to sample all areas of the breast mass.

EXCISIONAL BIOPSY – is the removal of entire breast mass under local anesthesia and sending of the specimen to the laboratory. The result takes 7 to 10 days to be available. Definitive removal of the entire mass is done. False negative absolutely none.

DEFINITIVE TREATMENT:

For CANCER – see section on CANCER

BENIGN TUMORS – see section on CYST AND TUMORS

BREAST PAIN + NIPPLE DISCHARGE (bloody) in a 25 YR OLD

Breast pain that is associated with a nipple discharge which is usually bloody occurs in a young girl whether she has borne children or not.

DIAGNOSIS: INTRADUCTAL PAPILLOMA

CAUSE: Formation of a pedunculated or non-pedunculated mass inside the tubbles of the breast.

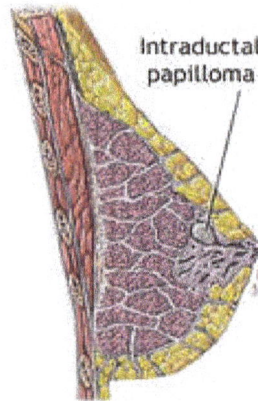

Common causes of abnormal nipple discharge

Intraductal papilloma

INITIAL TREATMENT: Pressure on the affected nipple and surrounding areas.

ADVICE:

Most bloody discharge in young women is due to a cyst like formation inside the tubes of the breast called PAPILLOMA. They are mostly benign and less likely to be malignant. They are often impalpable and difficult to locate by any diagnostic procedure. Biopsy may not be necessary but the fear of malignancy is still there.

LABORATORY EXAMINATION: none - no ancillary procedure could locate the mass.

DEFINITIVE TREATMENT:

EXCISIONAL BIOPSY – the nipple and the surrounding areas of the breast are milked towards the nipple to pinpoint the location of the duct. If the responsible duct is located, a wide incision is made following the course of the tube. The location of the papilloma is marked by a hematoma or pooling of blood in an area. A wide excision of the area is done to include all possible location of the papilloma.

HEADACHES

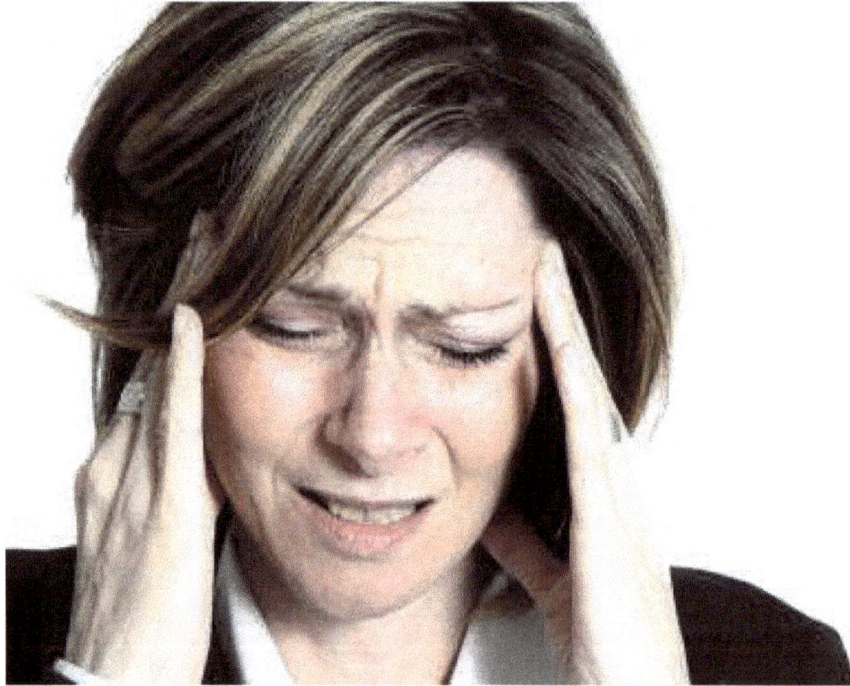

Common headaches are usually extra-cranial in origin and that is, they don't involve the brain. When they do, the symptoms are usually grave, namely; it is sometimes associated with weakness, tremors and dizziness, loss of consciousness or complete paralysis of the contralateral side of the body. As such, it could not be relieved by ordinary analgesics. Very often chronic and attacks would last for several hours.

Pinpointing the location of the headache gives the probable cause of the pain and the next possible steps to do to determine the cause. The objective here is to know whether to do further laboratory exams, consult a physician or submit to a suggested expensive diagnostic procedure. The reader is cautioned not to rely too much on his own "diagnosis" since other diseases may be masked by simple and mild symptoms but could be pathognomonic to a grave illness. Chronicity - is the prolonging of symptoms and an indication that the reader has to seek consultation.

FRONTAL HEADACHE

Headache noted on the frontal side of the face above the nose and in between the eyes usually throbbing aggravated by stooping down or bending forward. This is usually accompanied by a running nose in the early morning, stuffy nose in the evening and no symptom in the day. Cold weather initiates the symptoms but some maybe aggravated by hot climate. Some people may feel fullness on the sides of the nose and / or pain.

DIAGNOSIS: ACUTE SINUSITIS

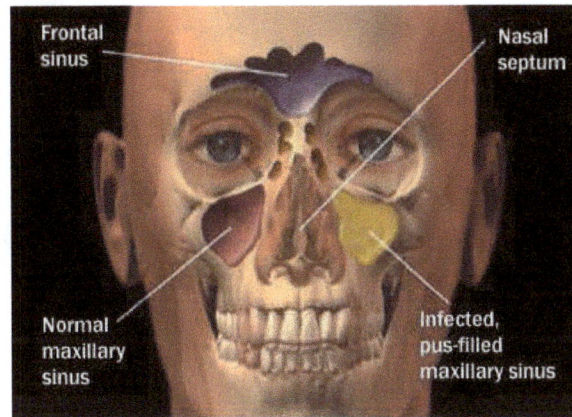

ORGAN INVOLVED: *Sinuses*

CAUSES:

ALLERGIES, such as allergic rhinitis that cause the swelling of the turbines inside the nose, are the initial problem. When this becomes lone standing, some of the mucus enters the sinuses (Sound chamber) found at the side of the nose and at the forehead and connected to the nose by inlets. When these become infected, swelling of the lining of the sinuses occurs.

COMMON COLD - blowing one's nose too hard causes the back-fire of mucus and infected elements into the sinuses.

INITIAL TREATMENT:

WARM WATER SHOWERS – no cold water showers in the morning and exposure to cold.

MENTHOL LINIMENTS - mix in warm water (Vicks Vaporub) they may open up clogged noses when inhaled. They must not be applied inside the nose nor eaten or chronically used.

ANALGESICS:
*MEFENAMIC ACID 500 mg tablet every 4 hrs **OR***
*DICLOFENAC NA 50 mg tablet every 6 hrs **OR***
PARACETAMOL 500 mg tablet every 4 hrs

DECONGESTANTS:
*NEOZEP tablet 3x a day **OR***
*DIMETAPP tablet 3x a day **OR***
NASATHERA tablet 3x a day

ANTIALLERGY:
*CETIRIZINE tablet daily **OR***
ZADEC tablet 3x a day (Ketotifen hydrogen fumarate)

ANTIBIOTICS:
*AMOXYCILLIN 500 mg 1 cap 3x a day **OR***
*TEQUIN 400 mg tablet daily for 3 days **OR (Gatifloxacine)***
*CLOXACILLIN 500 mg 1 cap 3x a day for 5 days **OR***
CLINDAMYCIN 300 mg 1 cap 3x a day for 1 week

ADVICE:

Treatment of headaches due to chronic sinusitis is geared towards the removal of infection, drainage of mucus from the sinus chambers, prevention of the recurrence of the allergy and keeping the sinuses open and clean. Due to the difficulty of achieving these objectives, no single treatment to this day, could possibly eradicate the symptom of headache in a Sinusitis sufferer. Thus, treatment objective is usually channeled to temporarily relieve the patient of symptoms of the current illness. Permanent cure is not expected.

DEFINITIVE TREATMENT:

DRAINAGE OF THE SINUSES – this is accomplished by actual pumping of the sinus chambers through the nose. The procedure is very uncomfortable and patient may feel like drowning.

INCISION AND DRAINAGE OF THE LATERAL CHAMBERS – making an incision inside the mouth thru the upper molars and drainage of the sinuses.

MIGRAINE HEADACHE

Severe headache on one side of the head usually preceded by an aura consisting of any or all of the following: halo formation around the light source, flushing the face, weakness, palpitations, pallor, numbness and tingling sensation of the teeth on the affected side of the face.

Migraine:
pain, nausea and visual changes are typical of classic form

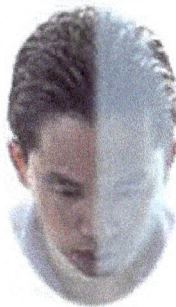

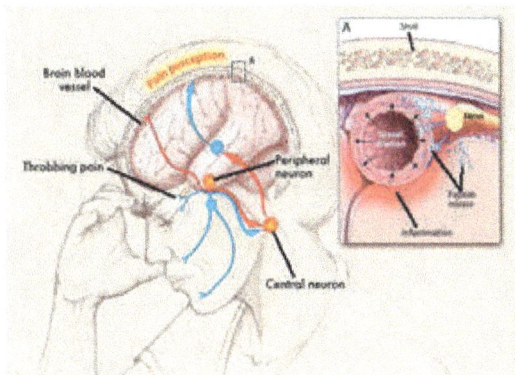

DIAGNOSIS: MIGRAINE

ORGAN INVOLVED: *nerves found in the scalp*

CAUSE: *Unknown* but severe factors have been noted to initiate migraine. PREVIOUS PSYCHOLOGICAL TRAUMA, PAST PHYSICAL TRAUMA, prolonged use of caffeinated products such as coffee, soft drinks, chocolate; exposure to chemical products and toxic fumes.

INITIAL TREATMENT: Cold showers and staying in cool places; removal and / or putting off loud noises. REST.

> *ANALGESICS: AVAMIGRAN tablet 3x a day* **OR**
> *MEFENAMIC 500 mg tablet every 4 hrs* **OR**
> *DICLOFENAC NA 50 mg tablet every 4 hrs.* **OR**
> *TRAMADOL 50 mg tablet every 12 hrs.*

ADVICE:

Most forms of treatment do not prevent further recurrence of pain. Avoidance of triggering factors and change of life style may help but do not assure absence of attacks.

LABORATORY EXAMS:

It is done to rule out the possibility of other disease entities like brain tumors: CT SCAN of the brain.

DEFINITIVE TREATMENT: *none*

STRESS PAINS

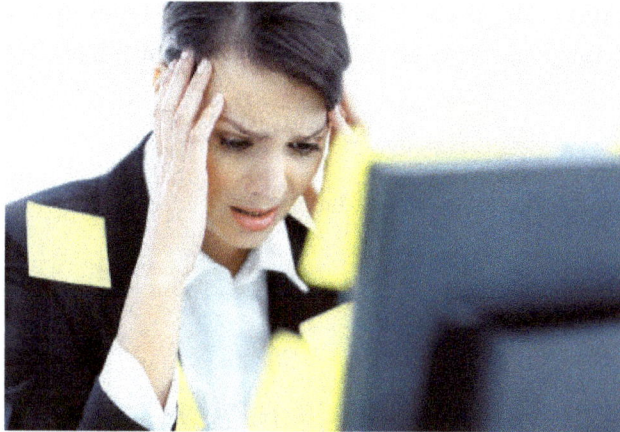

       Headaches due to stress are mostly and commonly generalized all over the head. But the most common point of pain complaints is at the temporal area. This may radiate to the scalp on top, at the side of the head, or at the forehead. This may be associated with head fullness or the feeling of heaviness in the head. Some people may experience dizziness, nausea, vomiting or even loss of consciousness.

DIAGNOSIS: STRESS HEADACHE

ORGAN INVOLVED: *brain*
CAUSE: STRESS
INITIAL TREATMENT: Sleep and getting away from the stressful circumstances are the best initial treatment for this kind of headache.
       ANALGESICS:

          MEFENAMIC ACID 500 mg tablet every 4 hrs. **OR**
          DICLOFENAC NA 50 mg tablet every 6 hrs. **OR**
          TRAMADOL 50 mg tablet every 12 hrs. **OR**
          ASPIRIN tablet every 4 hrs.

ADVICE:

A lot of headaches are due to job stress and / or situational stress. Cessation of exposure to the main cause of the headache treats the problem. Some people find relief in short relaxation. Others find consolation in psychotherapy, religion, sports and other activities, which deviate their attention away from the stress temporarily.

LABORATORY EXAM:

CT SCAN – use to rule out other cause of headache.

DEFINITIVE TREATMENT: *None*

PREAURICULAR PAIN

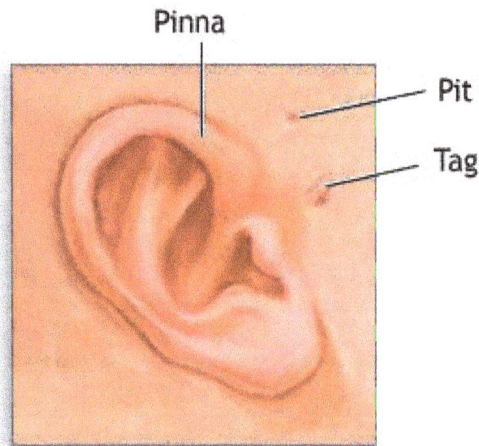

Pain located in front of the ear aggravated by opening the mouth associated with a grinding sound

DIAGNOSIS: ARTHRALGIA OF THE MANDIBULAR JOINT

ORGAN INVOLVED: bone joint of the mandible

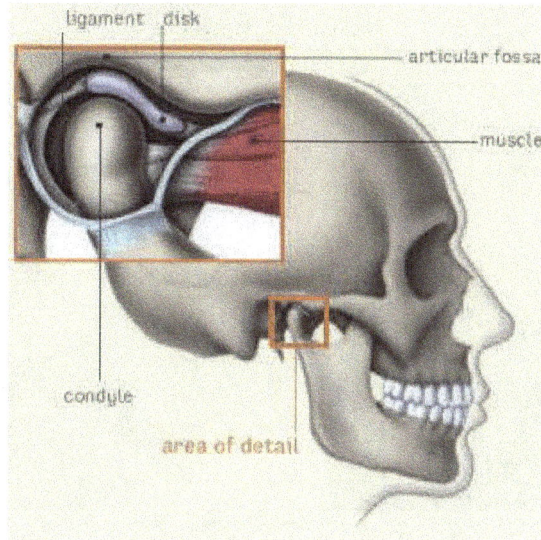

CAUSE: high uric acid; rheumatoid arthritis

INITIAL TREATMENT:

BEXTRA 50 mg tablet every 12 hrs. **OR***(Veldecoxib)*
ARCOXIA 120 mg once a day **OR (Etoricoxib)**
DICLOFENAC NA 50 mg tablet every 4 hrs.

ADVICE: Pains in these areas are usually found in older age group with a high uric acid in the blood. This is most often associated with other joint arthritis such as knee and elbow.

LABORATORY EXAMINATION:

X-RAY OF THE MANDIBLE - to determine if the bone joint is grossly affected.

URICACID DIET - examination of blood after fasting. (Post-midnight)

DEFINITIVE TREATMENT:

ALLOPURINOL 300 mg 1 tab daily for 3 months
PHYSIOTHERAPY

NUCHAL PAIN

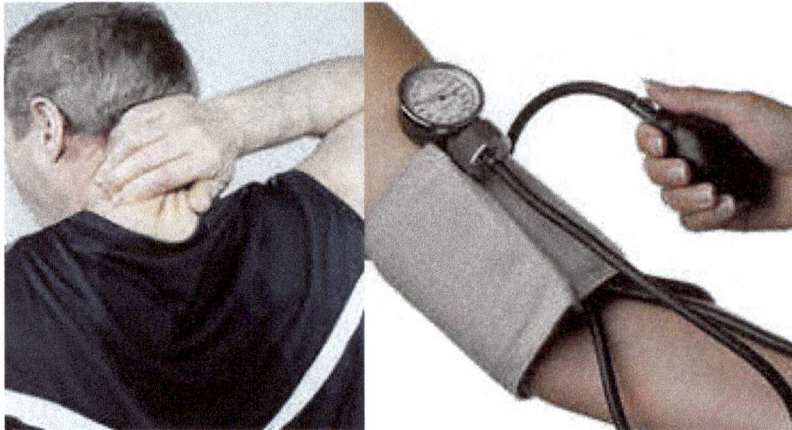

Pain felt at the base of the skull at the back of the head associated with head fullness, flushing of face, palpitation and dizziness.

DIAGNOSIS: HYPERTENSION

ORGAN INVOLVED: *Vascular system*

INITIAL TREATMENT: COLD COMPRESS on the face, chest, armpits, inguinal area.
TAKE BLOOD PRESSURE and let the patient recline or rest.

Give **ANALGESIC***: MEFENAMIC ACID 500 mg tablet every 4 hrs*

If known hypertensive, give anti – hypertensive even if patient has already taken his daily dose

ADVICE:
Nuchal pains are usually associated with hypertensive whose blood pressure has not been controlled by his / her medications. The pain is noted to be heaviness on the back of the head rather than pain per se and some would describe it as if a heavy object has been placed at the neck.

LABORATORY EXAMINATION:

LIPID PROFILE - determines cholesterol maybe one of the cause of hypertension.

CREATININE - to rule out the possibility of kidney failure causing hypertension

DEFINITIVE TREATMENT:

METROPOLOL 100 mg tablet daily or Losartan 50 or 100 mg daily

NEFIDIPINE 10 mg tablet daily or Amlodipine 5 or 10 mg daily

OCCIPITAL PAIN

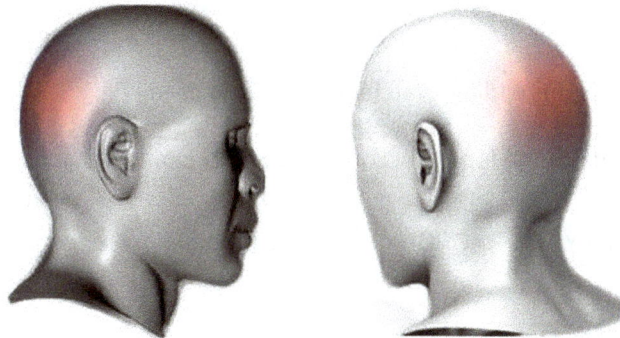

Pain at the back of the head exactly on the occipital prominence (pointed area at the back of the head) associated with blurring of vision, eye strain and / or glaring vision.

DIAGNOSIS: VISUAL DEFECT

ORGAN INVOLVED: *eye*

CAUSE: astigmatism, error of refraction, or cataract.

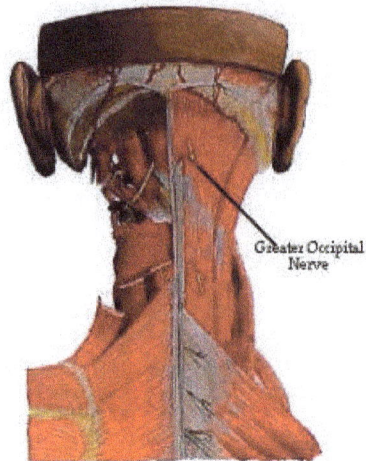

Greater Occipital Nerve

INITIAL TREATMENT: eye rest from reading, watching, television or movie.

ADVICE: The loss of the capacity of the lens to accommodate is the main reason for this problem.

LABORATORY EXAMINATION: EYE REFRACTION or eyeglass fitting

DEFINITIVE TREATMENT: *Eyeglass*
     Contact lenses
     Laser surgery

GENERALIZED HEADACHE

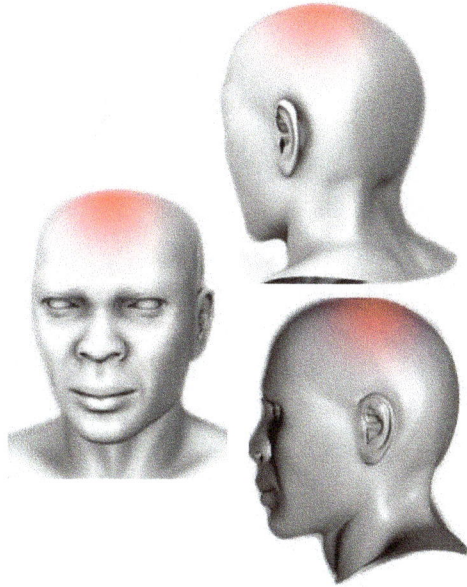

Headaches that could not be pointed specifically, but they are generally located at the side of the head above the ears and / or on top of the crown. This is associated with nausea / vomiting and generalized dizziness and the feeling of fullness of the headache. The pain is described as stabbing or crunching and could not be relieved by rest or sleep. Medications are sometime ineffective and attacks come at no specific interval and mostly occurring when the person is physically active. There is no neurologic deficit (paralysis or weakness of the extremities of side of the body) on examination. Spiking fever often accompany the symptoms.

DIAGNOSIS: ACUTE MENINGITIS

ORGAN INVOLVED: Brain Coverings: The Meninges

CAUSE: Bacterial Infection systematic in origin

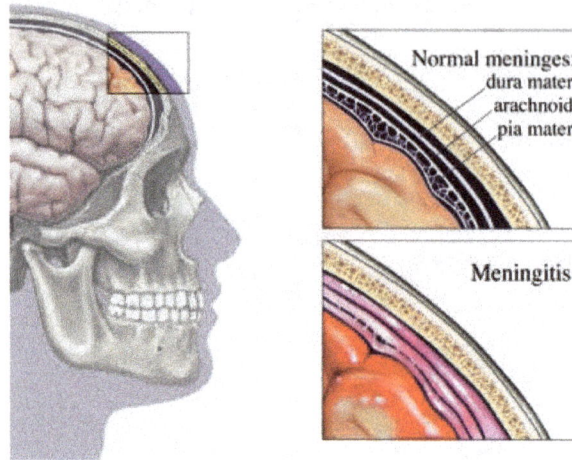

Normal meninges:
dura mater
arachnoid
pia mater

Meningitis

INITIAL TREATMENT: *none*

ADVICE:

Most often involved are children who had history if middle ear infection, spinal column injury, cranial injury, upper respiratory tract infection such as the nose and sinuses. Diagnosis is often missed due to latent symptoms and masked clinical signs. All children with history of headache should have a screening of possible infection of the meninges.

LABORATORY EXAMINATION:

LUMBAR TAP - aspiration of the brain fluid (CEREBROSPINAL FLUID) done at the back of the patient at the level of the lumbar vertebrae. Though the procedure is innocuous, accidental brain herniation may occur when there is a concomitant high cranial pressure. The fluid is brought to the laboratory to determine the presence of bacterial infection.

CT SCAN – used to determine meningeal swelling and rule out the possibility of tumors in the brain.

DEFINITIVE TREATMENT:

PARENTERAL ANTIBIOTICS – the patient has to be admitted for administration of potent antibiotics specific to the kind of bacteria present. This may be in the form of third generation cephalosporin, aminoglycosides, and third generation macrolides such as TEQUIN.

POSTAURICULAR PAIN

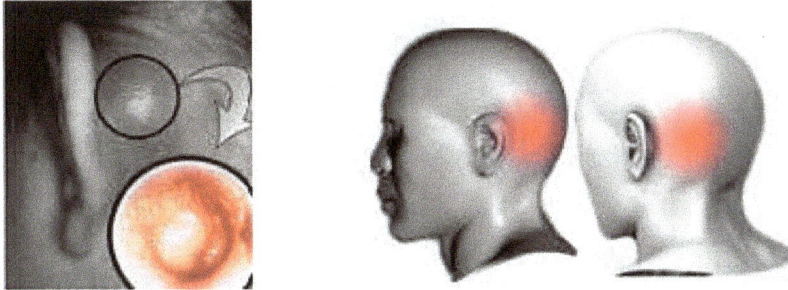

Pain at the back of the ear associated with swelling of the area and fever. A history of long standing middle ear infection is usually the case.

DIAGNOSIS: ACUTE MASTOIDITIS

ORGAN INVOLVED: bony prominence of the skull at the back of the ear. (MASTOID)

CAUSE: infection of the mastoid bone after a long – standing bacterial infection of the middle ear.

INITIAL TREATMENT:
    CLOXACILLIN 500 mg 1 cap 4x a day for 15-20 days **OR**
    CLINDAMYCIN 300 mg 1 cap 3x a day for 15 -20 days
    Cleaning of the ear: HYDROGEN PEROXIDE with the use of cotton tipped applicators.

ADVICE: Prevention of this illness is better than cure. Complete and proper treatment of ear infection prevents the onset of this disease.

DEFINITIVE TREATMENT:
    MASTOIDECOMY – it is the removal of the bony prominence at the back of the ear through proper debridement of the area by chiseling the pus – filled bone spaces. The patient is put under general anesthesia.

74

INFRA-AURICULAR PAIN

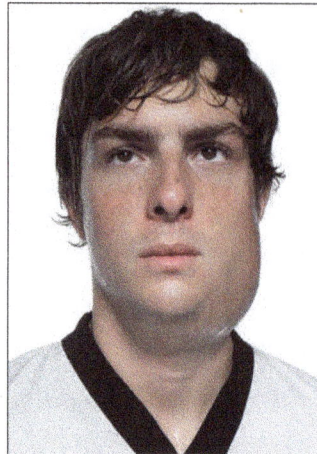

Pain occurring at the inferior side of the ear lobe radiating to the front, back and below the jaw aggravated by eating or drinking acidic foodstuff or citrus fruits and associated with high grade fever.

DIAGNOSIS: MUMPS

ORGAN INVOLVED: Parotid gland

CAUSE: Viral Infection of the Parotid Gland

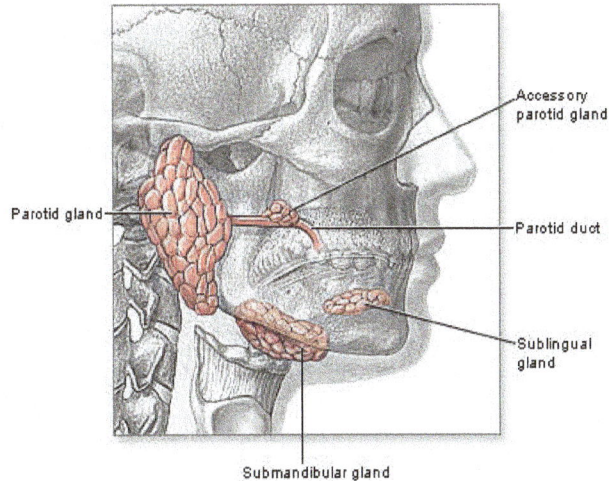

Parotid gland

Accessory parotid gland

Parotid duct

Sublingual gland

Submandibular gland

INITIAL TREATMENT:

PARACETAMOL 500 mg tablet every 4 hrs. **OR**
MEFENAMIC 500 mg tablet every 4 hrs.
AVOIDANCE of acidic and citrus fruits
Proper mouth hygiene

LABORATORY EXAMINATION: *none*

ADVICE:

Suppression of the high-grade fever is of utmost importance. Secondary involvement of the testes in males is possible and may progress into ACUTE ORCHITIS leading to sterility

DEFINITIVE TREATMENT:

VALTREX 500 mg *tablet* 3x a day for 10 days (Valaciclovir)

EXTREMITY PAINS AND NUMBNESS

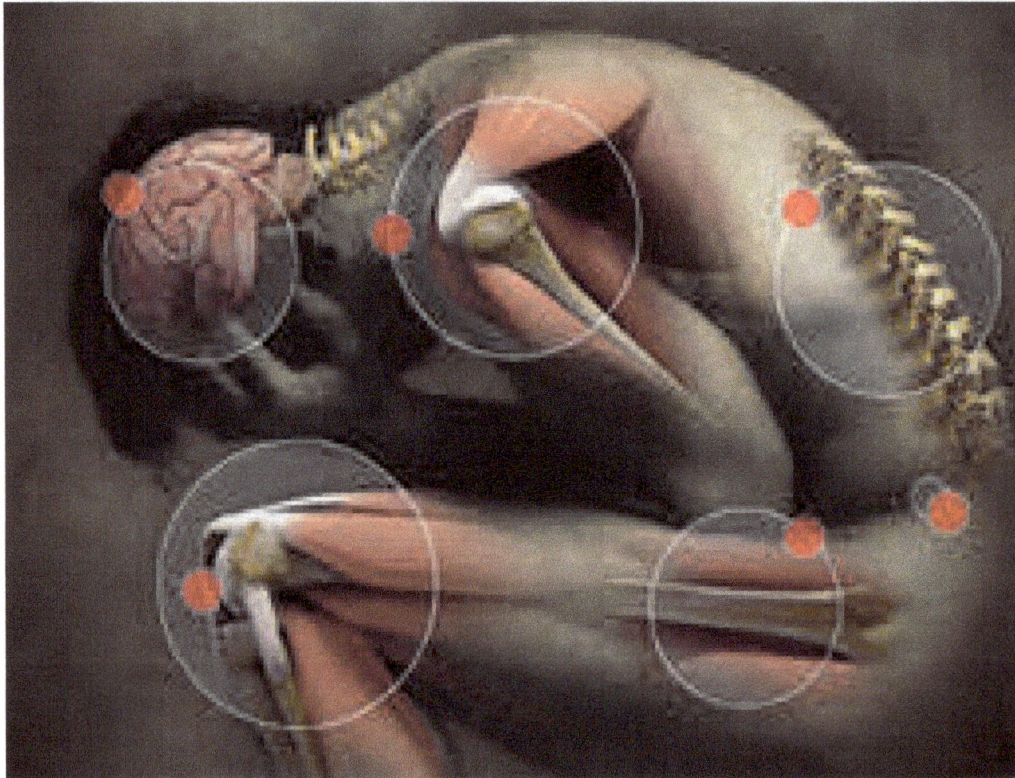

Pains in the extremities are most often due to sprains and fractures. But there are other illnesses in the extremities outside of the injury, which are very valuable to the sufferer in terms of knowing why they happen, its causes and where does it lead. Knowing the accompanying symptoms may help the sufferer pinpoint the culprit, and, what medicine to buy "over the counter" to ease the pain and what emergency procedures that should be done in order to prevent further damage to the affected area.

JOINT PAINS

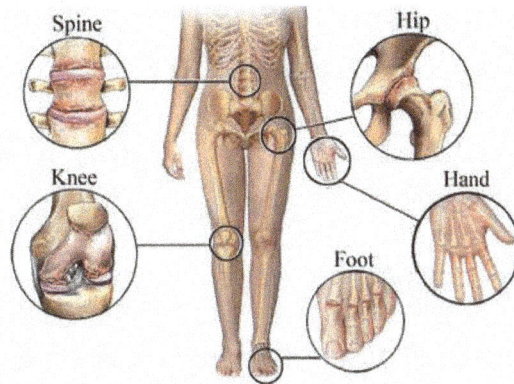

Pains in the joint usually occurring early in the morning or in cold weather associated with stiffening of the joints transferring from one joint to the other with no associated or history of trauma.

DIAGNOSIS: ARTHRITIS

ORGAN INVOLVED: bone joints

CAUSE:

Swelling of the lining of the bone joint (arthritis) or the bone joint itself (osteoarthritis). One cause is high uric acid in the blood. Other causes are unknown but usually afflict anybody above 35 yrs. old and above age group.

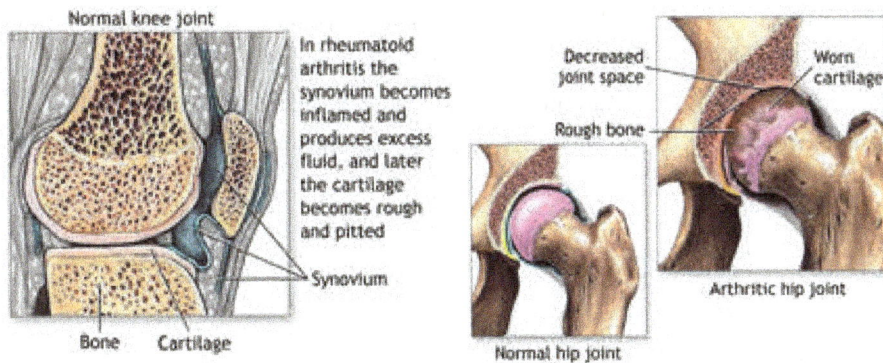

INITIAL TREATMENT:

Warm compress on the joints daily
IBUPROFEN 800 mg tablet daily OR
DICLOFENAC NA 50 mg tablet every 4 hrs. OR Stomach irritant
COLCHININE tablet 3x a day OR
CELECOXIB 200 / 400 mg tablet daily OR
ETORICOXIB 120 mg tablet daily OR
VALDECOXIB 40 mg tablet daily OR
ALLOPURINOL 300 mg tablet daily (for high uric acid blood determination)

BETHAMETHASONE JOINT INJECTION – intrathecal and usually done by physician. Relief may reach 2 - 3 months with possible kidney and liver complications.

ADVICE:

Most joint pains are only temporarily relieved by medications. No therapy has successfully terminated pains. Indications to do definite treatment are: extremely limited range of motion, severe pain limiting productive life and normal physical hygiene. There is no currently discovered preventive medicine.

LABORATORY EXAMINATION:

X-RAY OF THE JOINT – to determine damage but less helpful
MRI of the joint - most accurate examination to determine extent of damage.

URIC ACID DETERMINATION – may determine cause

DEFINITIVE TREATMENT:

COMPLETE JOINT REPLACEMENT - involving the replacement of the normal bone joint with composite made materials like titanium, ceramics, plastic resins, and stainless steel. This is a major surgery, which involves physiotherapy post-surgery, crutches for moths and instability for weeks.

TENNIS ELBOW

Arm in normal position.
Arms by side thumbs in.

Posterior / Back

Anterior / Front

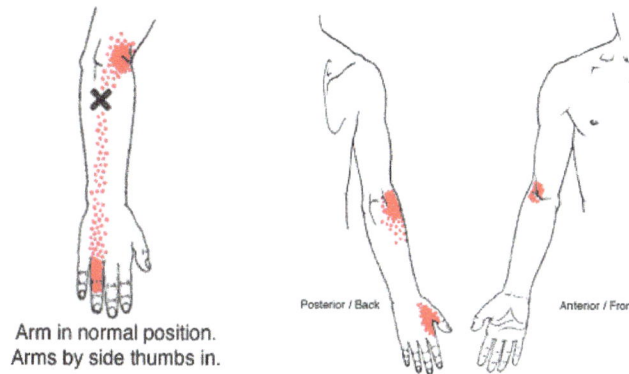

Pain on the elbow usually associated with abrupt and constant use of elbow in a short time such as in tennis playing, rowing, and other physical activity where the elbow joint is overworked.

DIAGNOSIS: ACUTE TENDINITIS

ORGAN INVOLVED: tendon attachments

CAUSE: straining of the muscle attachment to the elbow or bone joint

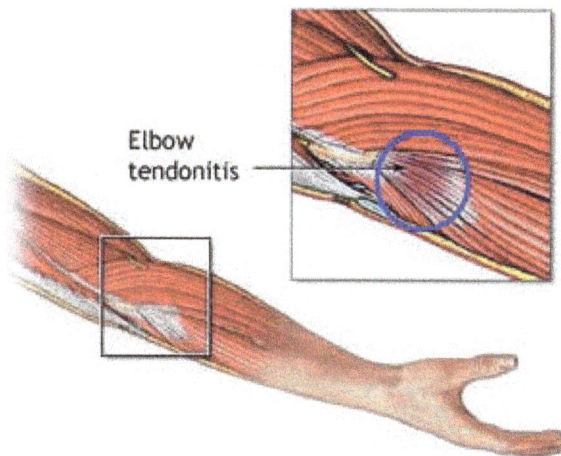

Elbow
tendonitis

INITIAL TREATMENT:

WARM COMPRESS ON THE ELBOW

ANALGESICS: MEFENAMIC ACID 500 mg tablet every 4 hrs. **OR**

DICLOFENAC NA 800 mg tablet daily **OR** *(Meloxicam 15 mg daily)*

IBUPROFEN tablet 3x a day **OR**

CELECOXIB 200 mg 1 cap 2x a day **OR**

ETORICOXIB 120 mg tablet daily

LABORATORY EXAMINATION:

MRI – is the most definitive diagnostic tool to determine other possible damage to the bone joint. Otherwise, it has negative findings.

X-RAY OF THE JOINT – not helpful

ADVICE:

Tennis elbow or accurate tendinitis is due to straining of the muscles found in the elbows. Abstinence or rest from the aggravating activity may give relief. Correction of the causative factor such as wrong swing as in golf or tennis may prevent recurrence of pain.

DEFINITIVE TREATMENT:

BETAMETHASONE INTRATHECAL INJECTION or on the site of pain - immediate relief of pain is usually accomplished.

PAIN AND NUMBNESS OF THE UPPER EXTREMITY

Pain associated with numbness of the upper extremity usually involving a portion or the whole arm or forearm extending from the axilla to the fingertips. Some people only experience the numbness component but others usually feel the pain described as pressure pain. Specific locations of the involved segments of the arm / forearm indicate the involved cervical neck involvement.

DIAGNOSIS: CERVICAL SPONDYLITIS

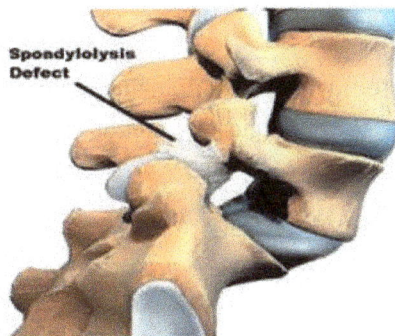

ORGAN INVOLVE: nerves coming from the neck supplying the upper extremity

CAUSE: VIRAL INFECTION OF THE PAROTID GLAND

INITIAL TREATMENT: calisthenics; physiotherapy of the neck
ANALGESICS: IBUPROFEN 1 tab 800 mg daily **OR**

CELECOXIB 200 mg 1 cap daily **OR**ETORICOXIB 120 mg 1 tab daily

NEUROTONICS: VITAMINS B complex1 tab 3x a day

ADVICE:

Pain and numbness of the upper extremity usually experienced by the elderly are caused by the impingement of the nerves exiting from the vertebra of the neck. This in turn is due to bone spicule formation that is similar to a wood stake hammered on top producing sharp pains. The cause of this formation is unknown but is usually found in people who carry heavy objects on their heads during their younger days.

LABORATORY EXAMINATION:

X-RAY OF THE CERVICAL VERTEBRAE – can view any or all aspects degenerative spondylitis

CT SCAN – specifically pinpoint the nerve involved and is necessary for contemplated surgery.

MRI - can magnify the possible involvement of the spinal cord

DEFINITIVE TREATMENT:

LAMINECTOMY – it is the removal of the impinging bone by surgery, which may lead to instability of the cervical vertebra. Newer surgical techniques remove this compromise.

SCIATICA

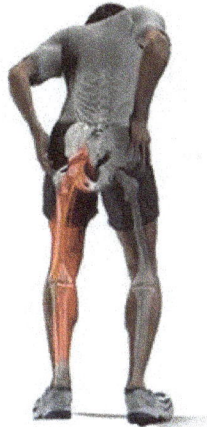

Pain originating from the back radiating downwards to the heel and is described as a shooting pain aggravated by standing up from a prolonged sitting position. Relief without medication is attained in a few minutes without treatment.

DIAGNOSIS: SCIATICA SECONDARY TO LUMBAR SPONDYLITIS
ORGAN INVOLVE: nerves exiting from the lumbar vertebrae

INITIAL TREATMENT: calisthenics; physiotherapy of the acupuncture

> *ANALGESICS: CELECOXIB 200 mg 1 cap daily OR*
> *ARCOXIA (Etoricoxib) 800 mg tablet daily OR*
> *IBUPROFEN tablet 3x a day*
> *NEUROTONICS: VITAMINS B $_1$– B$_6$ – B$_{12}$tablet 3x a day*

ADVICE: Most pains of this type are chronic in nature. Analgesics give temporary relief but do not remove the problem.

LABORATORY EXAMINATION:

X-RAY OF THE LUMBAR VERTEBRAE - will show the destroyed vertebrae in most cases showing degenerative changes.

CT SCAN – will show the specific nerve involved

MRI - will show the depth and extend of the problem

DEFINITIVE TREATMENT:

LAMINECTOMY - surgical removal of the impinging bone in the involved lumbar vertebrae thereby releasing the nerve affected. Instability of the vertebrae column may result. Long physiotherapy is necessary.

ANAL PAINS

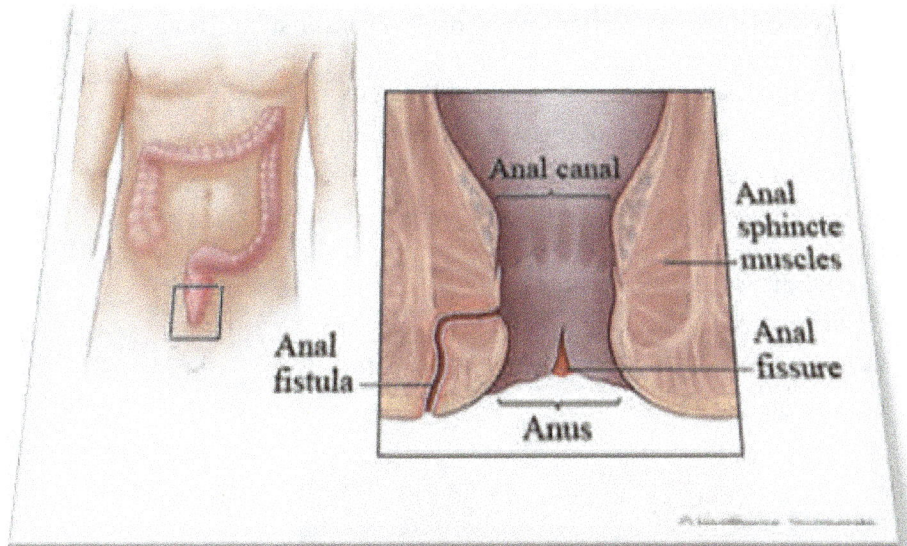

Anal pains are usually triggered by defecation. However, if there is an existing abnormality or disease, this may initially trigger the pain and cause further complications that could aggravate the pain. Since most anal pains are generalized and do not pinpoint the location of the problem, ocular inspection and digital examination are necessary. The following discussion is intended to give the reader the probable causes and their accompanying treatment before medical consultation is done.

ANAL PAIN AFTER CONSTIPATION

Pain experienced during bowel movement after several days of constipation. This is due to:

1. Fissures - small lacerations on the skin of the anus
2. Abrasions - partial removal of the skin of the anus
3. Laceration of preexisting hemorrhoids
4. Tagging of preexisting polyps in the anal verge

INITIAL TREATMENT – *hot sitz for 15 to 30 minutes*
FAKTU 1 Supp daily before going to bed
PROCTOGLYVENOL cream apply 2x daily with an applicator
DAFLON 1 tab 3x a day for 1 week

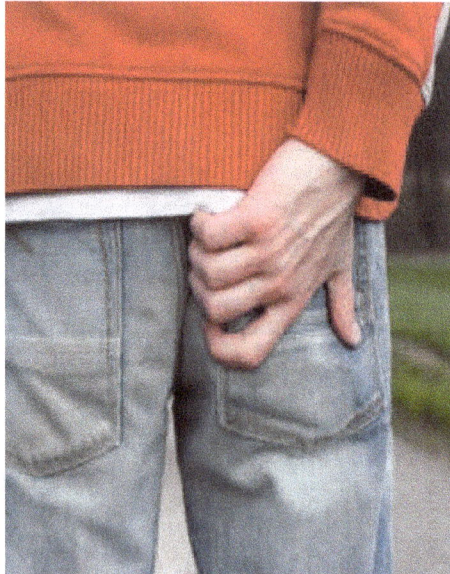

ADVICE: Most anal pains subside without treatment if there is no bleeding or laceration. Prevention is better than cure. Laxatives and intake of fruits produce soft stools (papaya, avocado, grape juice) these are recommended for people who are chronically constipated.

LABORATORY EXAMINATION:

PROCTOSIGMOIDOSCOPY – RIGID SCOPE – this is a half inch tube with a light source about 20 inches in length and inserted directly to the anus to visualize inner portion of the anus and the distal portion of the large intestine. It has a limited range and therefore it is not ideal to examine the whole of the large intestine.

COLONOSCOPY – FIBER OPTIC - this is done using a thin tube the size of the small finger, inserted into the anus and guided manually up to the whole length of the large intestine. Visualization is done through a TV monitor and/or thru the fiber-optic tube.

DEFINITIVE TREATMENT: correction of the disease.

PAIN AT THE ANAL SIDE

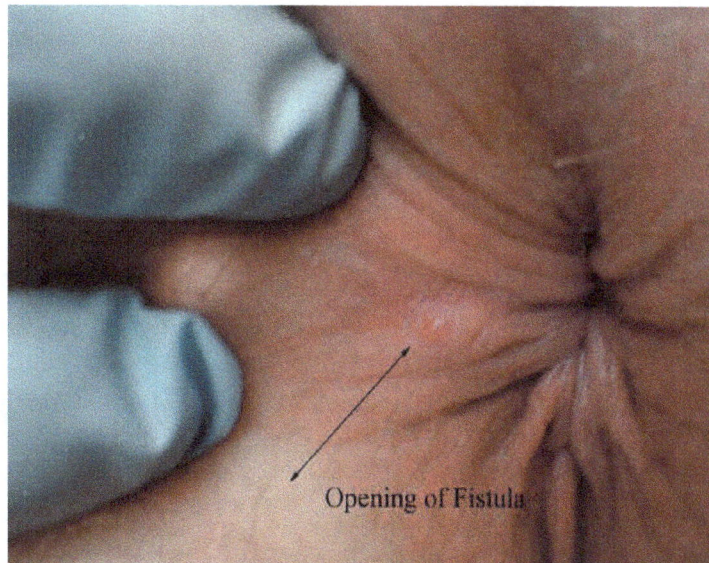

Opening of Fistula

This is a pain at the side of the anus accompanied by swelling. Formation of pus at or near the side of the anus that eventually becomes chronic despite antibiotic medications is visible.

DIAGNOSIS: FISTULA IN ANUS

CAUSE: tunnel formation from a pre-existing internal hemorrhoid

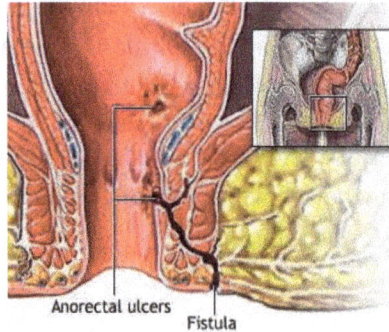

Anorectal ulcers
Fistula

ORGAN INVOLVE: skin of anal verge

INITIAL TREATMENT:

ANTIBIOTICS: CLOXACILLIN 500 mg 1 cap 4X a day for 7 day
METRONIDAZOLE 500 mg tablet 3X a day for 7days
ANALGESICS: MEFENAMICACID 500 mg tablet every 4 hrs.

ADVICE:

Untreated hemorrhoids cause canalization from the upper portion of the intestine down to the side of the anus. This is initially noted as a painful nodule that subsides with the intake of antibiotics but recurs after a few days. Subsequent recurrence will cause the formation of a small wound and the formation of a tunnel. Feces and liquid stools are channeled through this canal causing further swelling and abscess formation. Antibiotics do not close the canalization. Surgery is the only method of treatment.

LABORATORY EXAMINATION: rectal examination to determine the extent of the canalization. No x-rays of blood exam are necessary.

DEFINITIVE TREATMENT:

FISTULECTOMY - it is the removal of the entire length of the canal. Visualization of the canal is highlighted with the use of methylene blue solution. Excision of the entire canal is subsequently done. Recurrence is high if the fistulous tract is not completely removed.

FISTULOTOMY - opening of the roof of the canal and allowing it to close by itself (3 - 4 weeks). Recurrence is lesser through this method but unacceptable to the patient.

ANAL PAIN + BLEEDING + CONSTIPATION

Pain in the anus is triggered by the urged of defecation which is followed by a profuse bleeding of fresh blood after several days of constipation.

DIAGNOSIS: MALIGNANT LESION IN THE ANUS

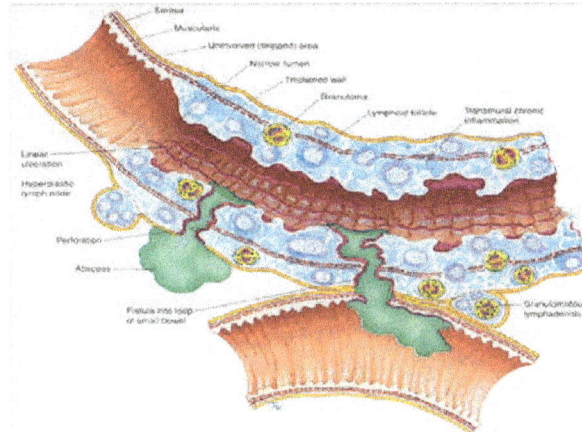

ORGAN INVOLVE: *rectosigmoid colon*

INITIAL TREATMENT: *none*

ADVICE:

Malignant lesions of the large intestine present in the different and non-specific symptoms: unexplained anemia, loss of weight, constipation, pragmatic loose bowel movement – constipation cycles, vague abdominal pains, odd anal discomfort, mucoid discharge, abdominal fullness and even chronic bleeding hemorrhoids. Routine examination of the anus must be done upon reaching the age of 35 yrs. old.

LABORATORY EXAMINATION:

RECTAL EXAMINATION – it is an examination of the anus with index finger. Minimal amount of discomfort most lesions are found through this simple examination.

BARIUM ENEMA – colonic cleansing with soapsuds is done the night before. An enema of whitish chemical is pumped into the anus with minimal pressure. Discomfort is felt when colon is full. Patient is asked not to discharge until procedure is fully accomplished. X – rays are taken on several positions and views

PROCTOSIGMOIDOSCOPY - a rigid instrument the size of a thumb and 20cm long is inserted into the anus. Visualization inside the anus is done directly with patient lying on his side. Discomfort is felt when the scope reaches the uppermost portion of the large intestine. Biopsy of any lesion found on examination can be done using long limbed pliers – like instrument called alligator forceps. No pain is felt but minimal bleeding may occur and blood can be noticed in stools for 24 hrs.

COLONOSCOPY – a flexible hose- like instrument the size of the small finger with light source of its own. The fiber optic cable is about 5 feet in length and can reach the uppermost portion of the large intestine. Visualization is done directly and thru TV monitor. Biopsy can be performed with this instrumental gadgetry.

CT SCAN – it is useful in determining the respectability, staging and spread (metastasis) of the tumor.

DEFINITIVE TREATMENT:

HEMICOLECTOMY - resection of the large intestine depending on the location of the tumor which could be right, left or transverse. Continuity of the intestinal tract is done thru end – to – end anastomosis (suturing). In some cases, due to difficulty of reattaching the intestines, the bowel segment brought outside thru a skin incision usually on the left side of the abdomen.

MILES RESECTION – is the removal of the intestinal tumor including the anus. Indicated in malignant tumors near the anus where continuity of the intestine is compromised. A permanent colostomy stump is made on the left side of the abdomen where the patient will subsequently move his bowel.

ANAL PAIN IN HEMORRHOIDS

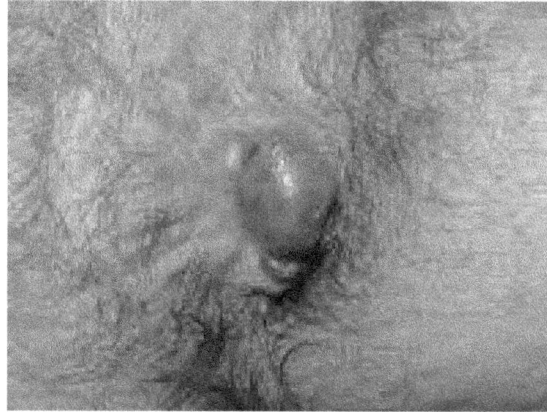

Pain in the anus associated with a mass dangling from the anal introitus, which may be triggered by several episodes of constipation, prolonged sitting down or irritation of the anus with the use of rough paper.

DIAGNOSIS: EXTERNAL HEMORRHOIDS

ORGAN INVOLVE: *anus*

CAUSE: pregnancy, lack of fluids in the diet, straining in bowel movement, straining in physical activity, heredity, unknown.

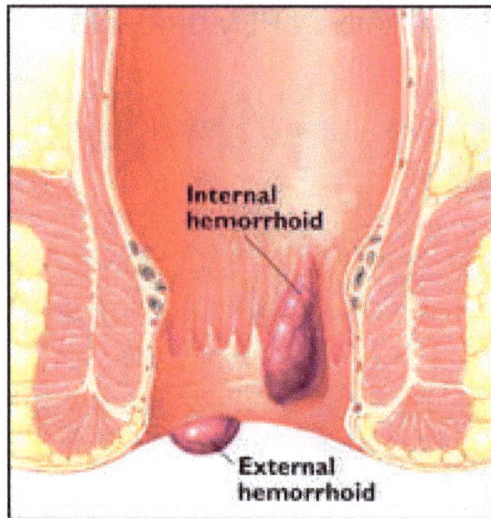

Internal hemorrhoid

External hemorrhoid

INITIAL TREATMENT:

HOT SITZ – sitting on a basin of warm water up to the level of the hips for 15 – 20 minutes 3x a day.

LAXATIVES:

SENOKOT (Senna - Rectal) GRANULES 1 tsp. daily **OR**

Dulcolax (Bisacodyl) tab 1 tab daily **OR**

DUPHALAC (Lactulose) sy 1 tab daily

ANALGESICS:

MEFENAMIC ACID 500 mg 1 tab every 4 hrs. **OR**

DICLOFENAC SODIUM 50 mg tablet every 4 hrs.

ANTI –INFLAMMATORY:

DAFLON 1 tab 3x a day for 7 days

ANAL CREAMS:

PROCTOGLYVENOL CREAM apply 2x a day

ANAL SUPPOSITORY:

FACTU supp 1 stick daily for 7 days

ADVICE:

Swelling of the hemorrhoids is the main cause of pain in the anus. Relief with the use of analgesic can be attained but recurrence is very common. Hemorrhoids can be conservatively treated for life. But with the onset of bleeding, swelling and thrombosis (clogged veins) surgery is indicated to prevent further complications like FISTULA IN ANUS.

LABORATORY EXAM:

BIOPSY OF THE HEMORRHOIDAL MASS – is necessary to screen out the possibility of malignancy presented by any anal mass such as hemorrhoids.

DEFINITIVE TREATMENT:

HEMMORRHOIDECTOMY:

WHITEHEAD TECHNIQUE – removal of the entire mass attached to the anus usually indicated for hemorrhoids that are extensive encompassing the whole diameter of the anus. Recurrence is very minimal. Hospital stay is prolonged. Bleeding post operatively may be great but do not require transfusion. Other posts of complications are:

WET ANUS -- exposure of the intestinal mucosa due to overextension of surgery which may happen when swelling is extensive prior to surgery. May last for months but could not recover. Anal discomfort is the main complain but may be alleviated with the use of diapers.

CONSTRUCTION OF ANAL CANAL – the hole of the anus may become small causing discomfort or pain on defecation. This may require dilatation under spinal anesthesia if bowel movement is greatly affected.

DIAMOND TECHNIQUE – piecemeal removal of the hemorrhoids with diamond shape incisions made longitudinal to the anal canal. No severe complications but recurrence is very high.

BACK PAINS

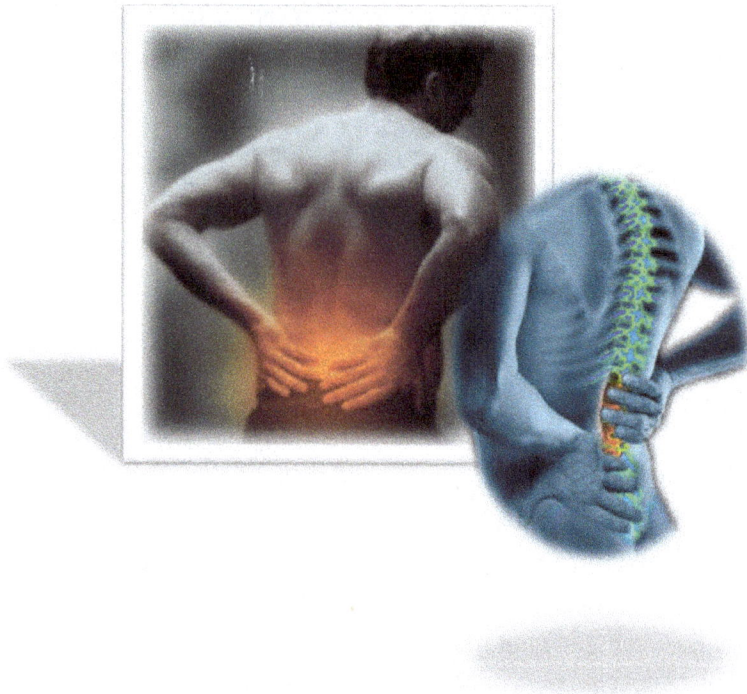

Back pains in general are caused by muscle spasms. Although some may originate from vertebral disease, most back pains originate from muscle strain, over fatigue, wrong posture or low calcium intake. Sudden change of physical activity from sedentary to hyperactivity or its opposite may cause severe back pains, as well as, increase in physical burden, such as weight lifting or sudden increase of work load or even with mental activity, may trigger back pains. There are instances, when some diet food can trigger back pains, like carabao meat and snake delicacies. Also, COMMERCIAL FURNITURES and clothes design invented by manufacturers without the ergonomic functions in mind can trigger back pains (spring bed, seat with low back rest, high heels, etc.)Eliminating or avoiding these causative factors may help in the treatment of the disease.

INTERSCAPULAR PAINS

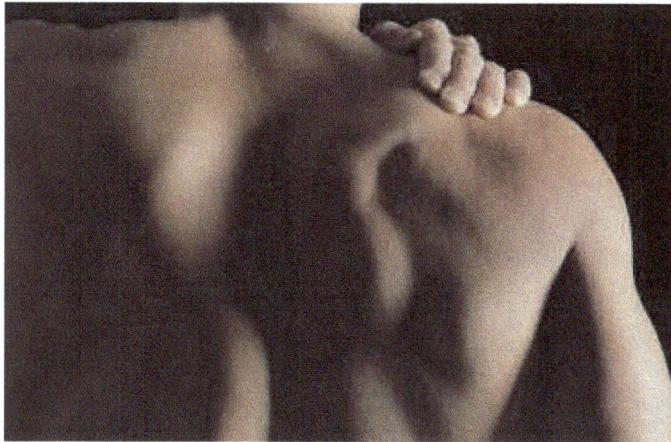

Pains located in between the scapula aggravated physical activity and usually relieved by light massage. There is no cough or any respiratory problem.

DIAGNOSIS: MYALGIA

CAUSE: muscle strains with excessive use of the right arm / forearm such as in sports or any household chores.

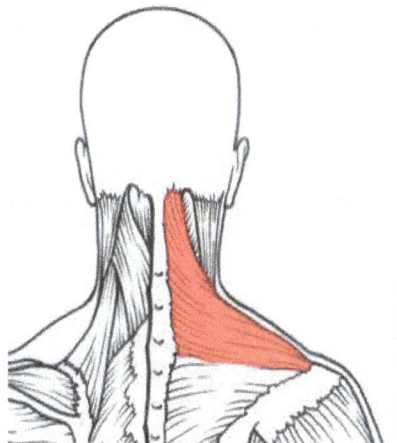

INITIAL TREATMENT:

MASSAGE: light massage using liniments

ANALGESICS: MEFENAMIC 500 mg 1tab every 4 hrs. **OR**

IBUPROFEN 100 mg tablets every 4 hrs.

MYONAL tablet 3x a day **OR**

NORGESIC tablet 3x a day

ADVICE:

Most pains in this area are due to muscle strain and are often secondary to sudden or rapid physical activity without warm up. Gradual increase of physical activity prevents occurrence. Without medication symptoms will abate in 5 to 7 days but will recur if physical activity is resumed.

LABORATORY EXAMINATION:

CHEST X-RAY – to rule out the possibility of lung diseases.

DEFINITIVE TREATMENT: *none*

TORTICULIS

Pain on the shoulder extending from the nap down to the shoulder tip aggravated by turning the head associated with rigidity of the muscle. This may often cause limitation of the range of motion such as turning the head left or right.

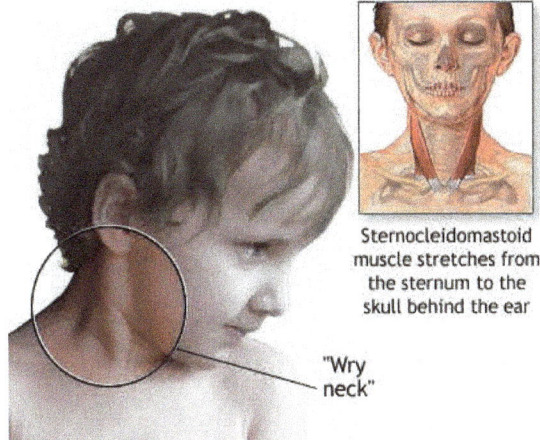

Sternocleidomastoid muscle stretches from the sternum to the skull behind the ear

"Wry neck"

DIAGNOSIS: TORTICULIS

ORGAN INVOLVE: muscles of the shoulder blade

CAUSE: *Hypocalcemia*

INITIAL TREATMENT:

Muscle Relaxants:

NORGESIC 1 tab 3x a day **OR**

ALAXAN tablet 3x a day

MYONAL tablet 3x a day OR

MEFENAMIC ACID 500 mg tablet every 4 hrs.

MASSAGE - with liniments

ADVICE:

Inadequate intake of calcium may lead to stiffening of the muscles most especially the muscles in the shoulder, neck and back. Fatigue due to over exercise, stressful physical activities and stressful mental activities may trigger symptoms

LABORATORY EXAMINATION:

SERUM CALCIUM DETERMINATION – a blood exam used to determine the level of calcium.

DEFINITIVE TREATMENT:

ESVICAL tablet daily **OR**
CALTRATE tablet daily **OR**
ONE tablet daily

BACK PAIN + COUGH +SMOKING

Back pains usually felt in the evening or early in the morning aggravated by cough found in a smoker. There may be loss of weight, coughing out of blood (hemoptysis) or nothing at all.
DIAGNOSIS: CANCER OF THE LUNGS

ORGAN INVOLVE: *lungs*

CAUSE: nicotine, highly suspected in most cases

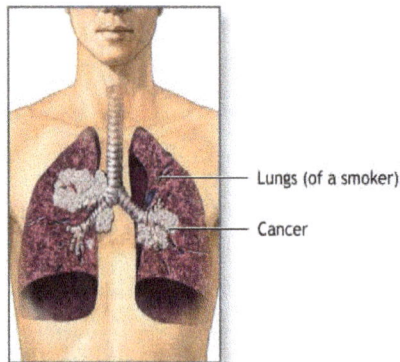

Lungs (of a smoker)

Cancer

INITIAL TREATMENT: STOP SMOKING

ADVICE:

There is a high incidence of lung cancer in smokers. Pathophysiology is not known. Diagnosis is followed by death in 6 months. Early diagnosis is rare. Late stage of discovery is the rule.

LABORATORY EXAMINATION:

CHEST X-RAY – suspicious lesions in the form of circular spots (cannon ball lesions) could be found on routine exam.

BRONCHOSCOPY – a tube is inserted direct into the lungs to determine the extent of the lesion for surgery. This diagnostic tool does not lead to early diagnosis. Bronchial washing may be detecting some of the early lesions.

CT SCAN of the THORAX – small lesions of lungs in their early stage could be detected. But routine examination with the use of this diagnostic stool is very expensive.

DEFINITIVE TREATMENT:

LOBECTOMY – total removal of the involved lobe of the lungs. This is indicated when the lung lesion is confined to one lobe of the lung. Otherwise, resection of the whole lung does not increase survival.

CHEMOTHERAPY OR RADIOTHERAPY - does *not increase survival.*

BACK PAIN + HISTORY OF TB

Back pains at the level of the thoracic vertebra between the scapular blades usually occur after work. No cough may be detected but most sufferers have history of lung tuberculosis. Extreme temperature and any stressful physical activity may aggravate the pain.

DIAGNOSIS: POTT'S DISEASE (TUBERCULOSIS OF THE SPINE)

ORGAN INVOLVE: Spine (Thoracic Vertebra)

CAUSE: Mycobacterium tuberculosis

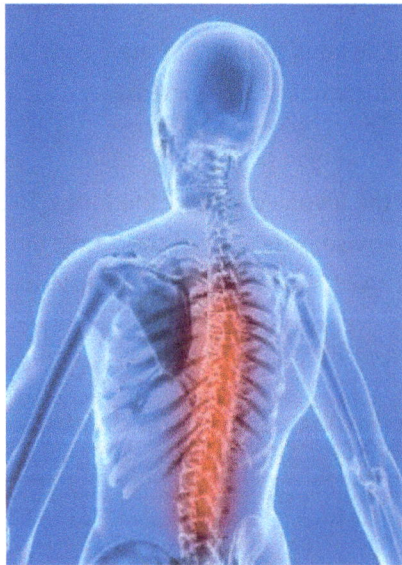

INITIAL TREATMENT
> *MEFENAMIC ACID 500 mg* tablet*every 4 hrs.* **OR**
> *DICLOFENAC NA 50 mg* tablet *every hour* **OR**
> *IBUPOFREN* tablet *every 4 hrs.*

ADVICE:

Tuberculosis may involve any part of the human body from the skin down to the bones. Incomplete treatment of the lung infection may lead to dissemination of the bacteria to other parts of the body. Because of the proximity of the THORACIC vertebra to the lungs and the common veins that drain these areas, transmission of the bacteria to the spine is very common.

LABORATORY EXAMINATION:

CHEST X-RAY – is applied to determine the primary focus of infection if it still exists.

X-RAY OF THE THORACICS VERTEBRA – determines the extent of the bone destruction and the necessity of surgery for the debridement and reconstruction.

CT SCAN OF THE SPINE - to determine the involvement of the spinal cord

DEFINITIVE TREATMENT:

ANTI – TB DRUGS: Multiple drug combination containing REFAMPICIN, INH, B_6, Pyrazinamine

ETHAMBUTOL

MYRIN P FORTE tablet 3x a day for 6 months **OR**

MOLECURE I 1 pack a day for 6 months to 1 year **PLUS**

STREPTOMYCIN 1 gm. in 3x a week in combination with oral medications

DEBRIDEMENT AND / OR RECONSTRUCTION OF THE SPINAL COLUMN

LOW BACK PAINS

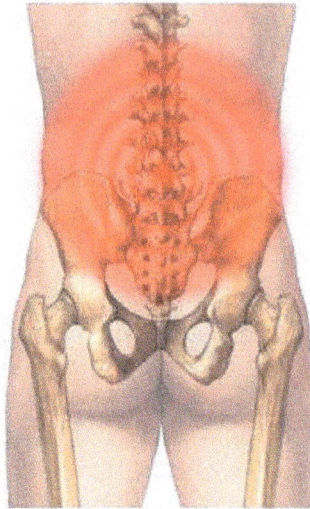

      Back pains at the level of the hips which usually occur after physical stress or even after a day's work radiating to the upper portion of the buttocks or involving the hip bones.

DIAGNOSIS: LUMBAGO / LUMBAR SPONDYLITIS

ORGAN INVOLVE: *lumbar vertebra*

CAUSE: stiffening of the lumbar vertebral column

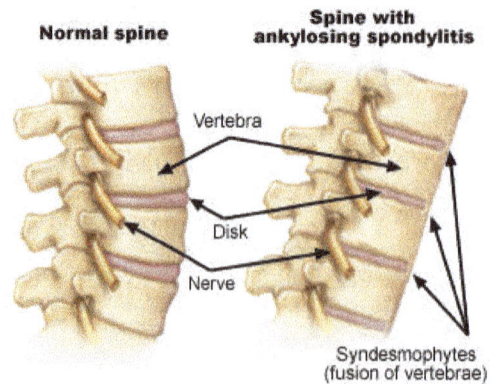

Normal spine

Spine with ankylosing spondylitis

Vertebra

Disk

Nerve

Syndesmophytes (fusion of vertebrae)

INITIAL TREATMENT

ANALGESICS:

MEFENAMIC ACID 500 mg tablet *3x a day every 4 hrs.* **OR**

ARCOXIA (Etoricoxib) 120 mg tablet *daily* **OR**

CELEBREX (Celecoxib) 200 mg 1 cap daily

CALISTHENICS - any exercise that could loosen the lumbar vertebral column such as turning the shoulder in opposite direction to the pelvis without moving the hips

MASSAGE / ACUPUNCTURE - claims of relief have been known.

ADVICE:

Back pain is usually due to improper posture in standing, sitting, lifting objects from the floor. Correction of these causes prevents further recurrence of the back pains. In older age group, the loss of vertebral pliancy as in lumbar freezing may be the main cause of the pain.

LABORATORY EXAMINATION:

X-RAY OF THE LUMBAR VERTEBRA – to determine the extent of stiffening of the lumbar bones and the presence of any spondylitic spike formation.

CT SCAN of the lumbar vertebrae - to determine the involvement of the spinal cord

MRI - can magnify the possible involvement of the spinal cord

DEFINITIVE TREATMENT: *none*

LOW BACK PAINS + SHOOTING PAINS TO THE LEGS

Pains in the back associated with shooting pain radiating to the foot per legs with numbness of the entire leg or crampy sensation most commonly aggravated by prolong standing or sitting.

DIAGNOSIS: SCIATICA

ORGAN INVOLVE: bone pressure on the spinal cord

CAUSE: displacement of the inter-vertebral disc (slipped disc) or pressure caused by vertebral spondylitis or formation of vertebral spicules secondary to age or trauma.

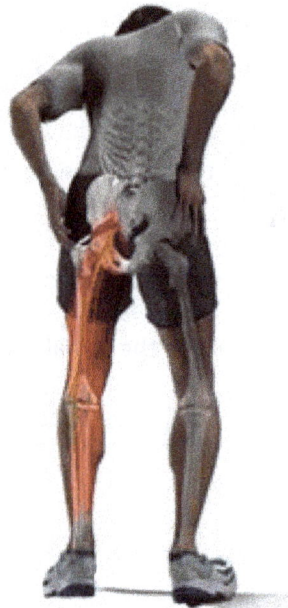

INITIAL TREATMENT:

ANALGESICS: BEXTRA (Valdecoxib) 50 mg tablet *daily* **OR**
ARCOXIA (Etoricoxib) 120 mg 1 cap daily **OR**
CELEBREX (Celecoxib) 200 mg 1 cap daily **OR**

PHYSIOTHERAPY
MASSAGE
ACUPUNCTURE

ADVICE:

With the presence of pressure on the spinal cord by the slipped disc or spicules of the vertebra, there is no permanent treatment outside the surgery. However, complications of surgery may lead to permanent incapacity and more likelihood of disability. Treatment must be weighed before embarking on treating the disease.

LABORATORY EXAMINATION:

X-RAY OF THE LUMBAR VERTEBRAE may show the vertebral spicules but not help in the specific treatment

CT SCAN – it is the most specific diagnostic exam to visualize the affected spinal cord. This examination is both diagnostic as well as a mapping procedure to approach the problem surgically. It shows the axial view of the spinal cord.

MRI - some surgeons prefer to do this procedure in order to map out the involvement of the other areas of the spinal cord since it shows the longitudinal aspect of the spinal cord.

DEFINITIVE TREATMENT:

LAMINECTOMY – surgical removal of the involved vertebral part pressing on the spinal cord. Due to the vague boundary of this procedure (whether it is expertise of the neurosurgeon or orthopedic surgeon), the patient is cautioned as to what specialized treatment to select.

PAIN DURING URINATION

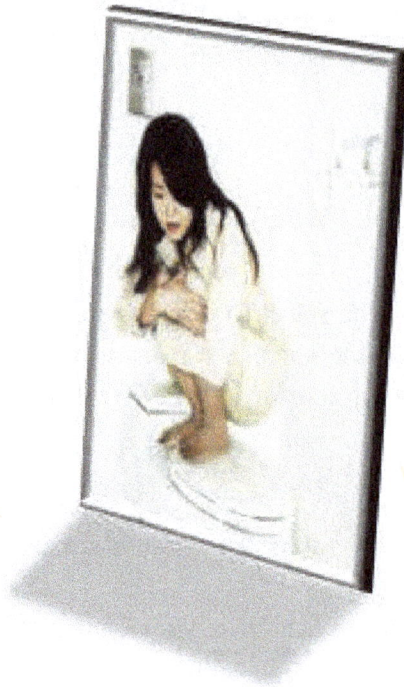

Pain initiated by the act of urination lasting up to the duration of the act most commonly described as burning, difficulty of urination, and / or there is blockade. This feeling is usually felt at the distal portion of the penis and / or in the middle of the penile shaft. There may be penile discharge of greenish material or none at all. Milking of the penile shaft may initiate the appearance of the discharge.

DIAGNOSIS: GONOCOCCAL URETHRITIS

ORGAN INVOLVE: *penis*

CAUSE: gonorrhea

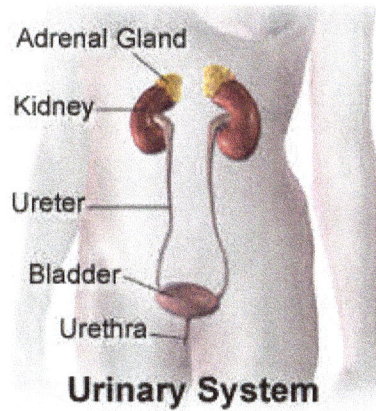
Urinary System

INITIAL TREATMENT: none

ADVICE:

Sexual intercourse is the only mode of transmission. Complete treatment is necessary to prevent recurrence and resistance of the bacteria. Prevention with the use of condom, washing, post intercourse urination, pre-intercourse antibiotics may help. Some of the recommended pre-intercourse preventive antibiotics are:

TEQUIN (Gatifloxacin) 400 mg tablet *before sexual intercourse* **OR**
CIPROBAY (Ciprofloxacin) 500 mg tablet*1 hr before sexual intercourse*
CEFUROXIME 500 mg tablet *before sexual intercourse*

LABORATORY EXAMINATION:

URETHRAL SMEAR – placing smudge of the discharge on a glass slide by touching its surface on the penile opening. It is positive when the bacteria are found inside the cells.

URINALYSIS – only indicates urinary tract infection without identifying the bacteria

DEFINITIVE TREATMENT:

TEQUIN (Gatifloxacin) 400 mg tablet daily for 5 days **OR**
CIPROFLOXACIN 500 mg tablet 2x a day for 7 days **OR**
CEFUROXIME 500 mg tablet 2x a day for 1 week

PAIN DURING URINATION WITHOUT DISCHARGE

Pain during urination similar to gonococcal urethritis but without the greenish discharge.

DIAGNOSIS: NON – GONOCOCCAL URETHRITIS

ORGAN INVOLVE: *penis*

CAUSE: E. coli, Chlamydia, Doderline bacillus, and other hosts of bacteria

INITIAL TREATMENT: *none*

ADVICE:

Infection of the penis could come from other sources outside sexually transmitted disease. Doderline bacillus, normal resident bacteria of the vagina may cause irritation to the penis post coitus (most common in honeymoon situations) penile contact of dirty surfaces such as toilet bowls and urinals may also cause infection.

LABORATORY EXAMINATION:

URETHRAL SMEAR – to determine the causative bacteria for the selection of the antibiotics
URINALYSIS – is applied to determine the extent of the urinary tract infection and duration of antibiotics.

DEFINITIVE TREATMENT:

TEQUIN (Gatifloxacin) 400 mg 1 tab single dose **OR**
CIPROFLOXACIN 500 mg 1 tab 2x a day for 5 days **OR**

PAIN IN THE NECK DURING SWALLOWING

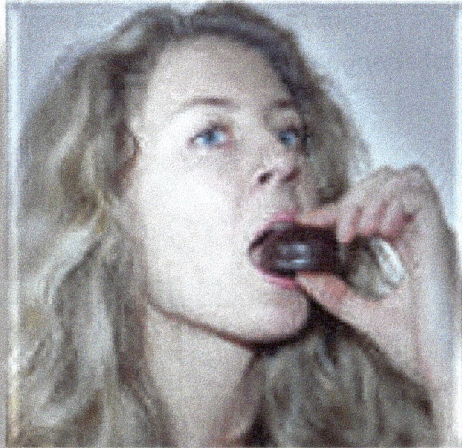

In general, pain in the neck is most often due to infection. Seldom do tumors and new growths in the neck are discovered prior to the pain experienced by the patient. They are primarily discovered as tumors and the pain comes later on. Thus, symptoms associated with or preceding pain are of utmost importance for the diagnosis. Treatment is based on what particular bacteria are responsible. Laboratory examinations are necessary when symptoms do not abate after several courses of treatment. However, X-ray modalities and imaging procedures are seldom necessary. And if they are needed, the doctor perhaps, entertains the possibility of underlying tumor or malignant new growth.

In particular, foreign bodies and fish bones that are stuck in the throat may also cause pain in the neck. The option whether to seek medical help or not lies in the perception of the patient whether his or her medication is adequate or not and the patient must wait for treatment to take effect. For immediate relief, nothing is faster than to seek medical attention.

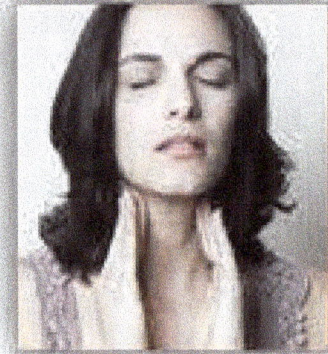

Thus, the objective of this chapter is to enable the reader to delineate which pain in the neck needs immediate medical attention and which pain a person can self-medicate.

SORE THROAT

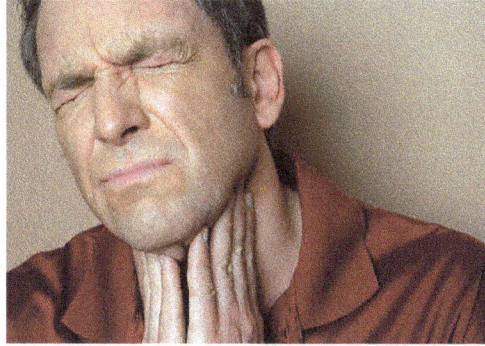

Pain in the throat is associated in the act of swallowing aggravated by food or fluid intake associated with fever and cough but NO COLDS.

DIAGNOSIS: BACTERIAL TONSILLO - PHARYNGITIS

ORGAN INVOLVE: tonsils and pharynx (back wall of the throat)

CAUSE: Streptococcal infection

INITIAL TREATMENT:

> *RITEMED AMOXYCILLIN 500 mg 1 cap 3x a day for 7 days* **OR**
> *CLOXACILLIN 500 mg 1 cap 3x a day for 5 days* **OR**
> *STREPSIL LOZENGES / DIFFLAM LOZENGES*
> *BACTIDOL MOUTHWASH*

ADVICE:

Most sore throats respond to ordinary antibiotics or even regular mouthwash. What is important is the frequency of the infection. If the sore throat becomes more frequent (more than 4x a year), the likelihood of having streptococcal infection leading to RHEUMATIC HEART DISEASE should be borne in mind.

LABORATORY EXAMINATION:

ASO TITER – blood examination to determine whether the sore throat infection may lead to RHEUMATIC HEART DISEASE

GRAM STAINING OF THROAT – throat swab done on the pharynx to isolate the bacteria responsible.

CULTURE AND SENSITIVITY – lab exam isolates the bacteria and determines the antibiotic most effective against it. This is most frequently necessary when the infection is resistant to common treatment and the symptoms persists despite adequate antibiotics

DEFINITIVE TREATMENT:

The cure is based on the isolated bacteria found in the CULTURE AND SENSITIVITY.

SORE THROAT + COLDS

Pain in the throat associated with body malaise, colds, fever, and cough. Some patients experience muscle pains and general lethargy.

DIAGNOSIS: ACUTE INFLUENZA

ORGAN INVOLVE: nose, throat bronchus, lungs

CAUSE: Viral Infection

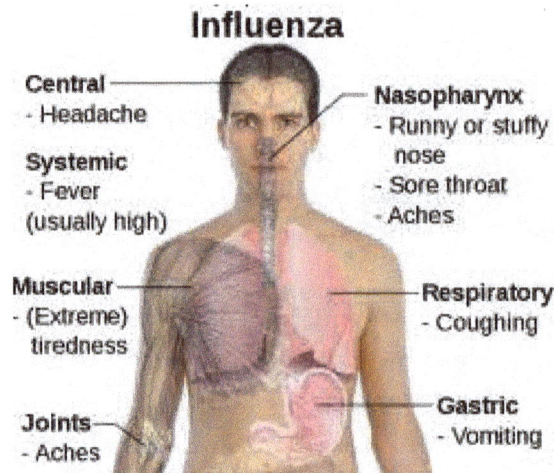

Influenza

Central
- Headache

Systemic
- Fever
(usually high)

Muscular
- (Extreme)
tiredness

Joints
- Aches

Nasopharynx
- Runny or stuffy nose
- Sore throat
- Aches

Respiratory
- Coughing

Gastric
- Vomiting

INITIAL TREATMENT:

    DECONGESTANTS: NASATHERA 1 tab 3x a day
    ANTIPYRETICS: PARACETAMOL 500 mg tablet every 4 hrs.
    ASPIRIN tablet every 4 hrs.
    PAIN RELIEVERS: MEFENAMIC 500 mg tablet every 4 hrs.
    COUGH SYRUPS:
    SINECOD 1 tbsp. 3x a day

ADVICE:

Most viral infection is self-limiting disease that means the symptoms subside without medications except for the symptom relievers. Thus, antibiotics do not have a role in the management of this illness. Complete bed rest, massage, keeping warm are all the things one needs to recuperate in 5 to 7 days.

LABORATORY EXAMINATION: *none*

DEFINITIVE TREATMENT:

If complications set in such as pneumonia, antibiotics are then necessary. Pneumonia heralded by difficulty of breathing, persistence of fever and severe cough with yellowish phlegm.

SORE THROAT + ACUTE HOARSENESS

This is a pain in the throat with fever and change of the voice. This may be preceded by colds and associated with cough.

DIAGNOSIS: NON – ACUTE LARYNGITIS

ORGAN INVOLVE: larynx

CAUSE: Bacterial infection

INITIAL TREATMENT:

    Warm infection, Warm soup, Warm drinks, Lozenge

ADVICE:

Most common colds result to superimposed bacterial infection when it involves the larynx or voice box. This occurs 3 to 5 days after the onset of the upper respiratory tract infection. When over the counter treatment does not afford relief, this is possibly due to bacterial laryngeal infection. The use of antibiotics is necessary when hoarseness set in.

LABORATORY EXAMINATION:

CHEST X-RAY – is a necessary step when cough becomes paroxysmal and persistent.

DEFINITIVE TREATMENT:

CLOXACILLIN 500 mg 1 cap 3x a day for 7 days
AMBROXOL 75 mg 1 cap once a day for 7 days

SORE THROAT + CHRONIC HOARSENESS

Sore throat associated with changes of the voice without colds or fever lasting for several weeks or even months.

DIAGNOSIS: NON – LARYNGEAL TUMOR

ORGAN INVOLVE: *larynx*

CAUSE: tumor or mass forming at the larynx or voice box.

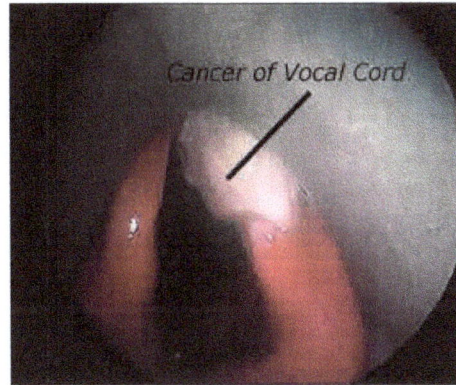

INITIAL TREATMENT: *none*

ADVICE:

Tumors of the larynx are sometimes symptomless. Change of the voice that the patient alone can only notice may be the only clue of its presence. The smaller they are, the better and easier the management. Malignant tumors require radical surgery to stop the rapid spread of the cancer but overall survival rate is dismal.

LABORATORY EXAMINATION:

LARYNGEAL BIOPSY OF THE TUMOR this requires bronchoscopy where a tube is inserted directly to the throat and the mass remove by a long instrument. This is then brought to the laboratory for microscopic examination. Anesthesia is local spray and does not usually require general for some patients.

CT SCAN OF THE NECK – this is required to determine the extent or possible spread of the tumor since this disease rapidly spreads to the nearby structures and to determine the extent of surgery.

CHEST X-RAY – done to determine the spread of the tumor to the lungs.

DEFINITIVE TREATMENT:

TOTAL LARYNGECTOMY – total removal of the voice box by surgery. A hole is made at the base of the neck where the distal remaining tube of the bronchus is attached and where the patient will now breathe (TRACHEOSTOMY).

CHEMOTHERAPY – prolongs life to 2 – 3 years.

COBALT TREATMENT - destroys tumors spreading near the voice box and adds more years.

DIFFICULTY OF SWALLOWING + FEVER

It is a pain that occurs during swallowing of solid food. This is preceded by sore throat, fever and sometimes colds.

DIAGNOSIS: ACUTE TONSILLITIS

ORGAN INVOLVE: tonsils

CAUSE: enlargement of the tonsils secondary to bacterial infection

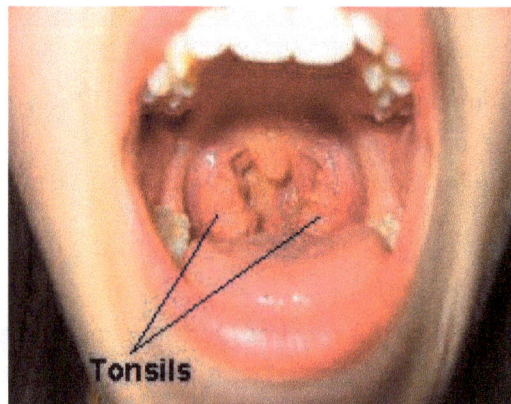

Tonsils

INITIAL TREATMENT:

CLOXACILLIN 500 mg 1 cap 3x a day for 7 days

BACTIDOL MOUTHWASH 3x a day

ADVICE:

Enlargement of the tonsils may be due to prolong or recurrent infection of the tonsils. Inadequate usage or under dosage of antibiotics may also be the cause. Prior to the discovery of good antibiotics, removal of the tonsils by surgery had been recommended.

LABORATORY EXAMINATION:

CULTURAL AND SENSITIVITY OF THE THROAT – is necessary when infection does not respond or subside with ordinary antibiotics. This only requires swabbing of the tonsils with cotton swabs and is not painful.

DEFINITIVE TREATMENT:

TEQUIN (Gatifloxacin) 400 mg *tablet* once daily for 3 days

DIFFICULTY OF SWALLOWING + NO FEVER

It is a gradual difficulty of swallowing solid foods. This may be initiated by frequent choking with difficulty of swallowing bigger sized foodstuffs. The patient initially feels no pain but there may be chest tightness.

DIAGNOSIS: ESOPHAGEAL CANCER

ORGAN INVOLVE: ESOPHAGUS (tube that carries food from the mouth to the stomach)

CAUSE: High incidence in person with Chinese descent. *Unknown*

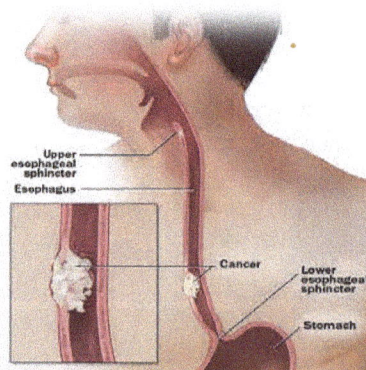

INITIAL TREATMENT: *none*

ADVICE:

Early diagnosis is of primary importance. Spread of cancer to other parts of the body defeats further radical treatment. Survival rate in patients with metastasis (spread) is dismal. The purpose of surgery rate is to preserve the continuity of the intestinal tract. Complications of post-surgery are very high and cost is prohibitive.

LABORATORY EXAMINATION:

GASTROSCOPY – visualization of the esophagus through a fiber-optic machine and concomitant biopsy of the mass or stricture is done.

ESOPHAGOGRAM – x-ray procedure whereby the patient is asked to swallow milky substance and x-ray is taken in the act of swallowing. This may visualize stricture or mass inside the esophagus. It is not a diagnostic in terms of determining malignancy.

DEFINITIVE TREATMENT:

ESOPHAGECTOMY - total removal of the esophagus from the base of the mouth to the stomach through an incision on the side of the chest. Continuity of the intestine is made by using a segment of the large intestine as esophagus or a portion of the stomach fashioned into a tube and attached to the remaining portion of the throat.

Some surgeons may opt for feeding of the patient through a tube inserted direct to the stomach (GASTROSTOMY TUBE FEEDING).

SWALLOWED COINS

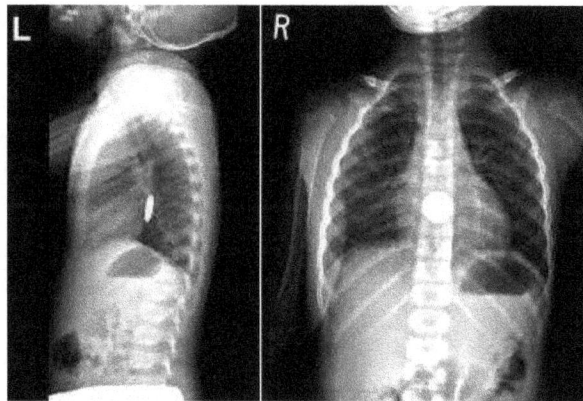

Most swallowed coins end up in the stomach and passed through the stools. But when the child has difficulty of breathing, the voice becomes hoarse or a gurgling sound could be heard when he / she breathes; the child should be rushed to the hospital.

DIAGNOSIS: FOREIGN BODY IN THE BRONCHUS

ORGAN INVOLVE: BRONCHUS – air pipe

INITIAL TREATMENT:

Calm the patient by giving him candy. NO WATER OR ANY SOLID FOOD. If the patient keeps on vomiting, let foodstuff come out without obstruction to prevent food from entering the air pipe. Do not attempt or coax patient to spit the coin.

ADVICE:

Patient has to be sedated in order to remove the coin by bronchoscopy. If stomach is full, the danger of food regurgitation into the lungs is high. Thus, a tube is usually inserted into the nose prior to the procedure of removing the coin from the bronchus. Infection after removal of the coin follows and may lead to bronchopneumonia. Bronchospasm (rigidity of the bronchus) may also occur. Thus, admission to the hospital is necessary for observation.

LABORATORY EXAMINATION:

CHEST X-RAY – to know the location of the coin whether esophagus or bronchus by mere chest x-ray is pinpointed by how the coin lies. If the coin is viewed as standing thin on its side, it is inside the bronchus. If flat on its face, it must be inside the esophagus. This is the fastest way to determine location.

BRONCHOSCOPY – patient is sedated or generally anesthetized. A tube is inserted through the nose into the stomach to prevent regurgitation of food into the lungs. A fiber-optic tube is directly inserted into the bronchus and a long forceps grasps the coin.

DEFINITIVE TREATMENT:

BRONCHOSCOPY – as described above

PAIN IN THE EAR

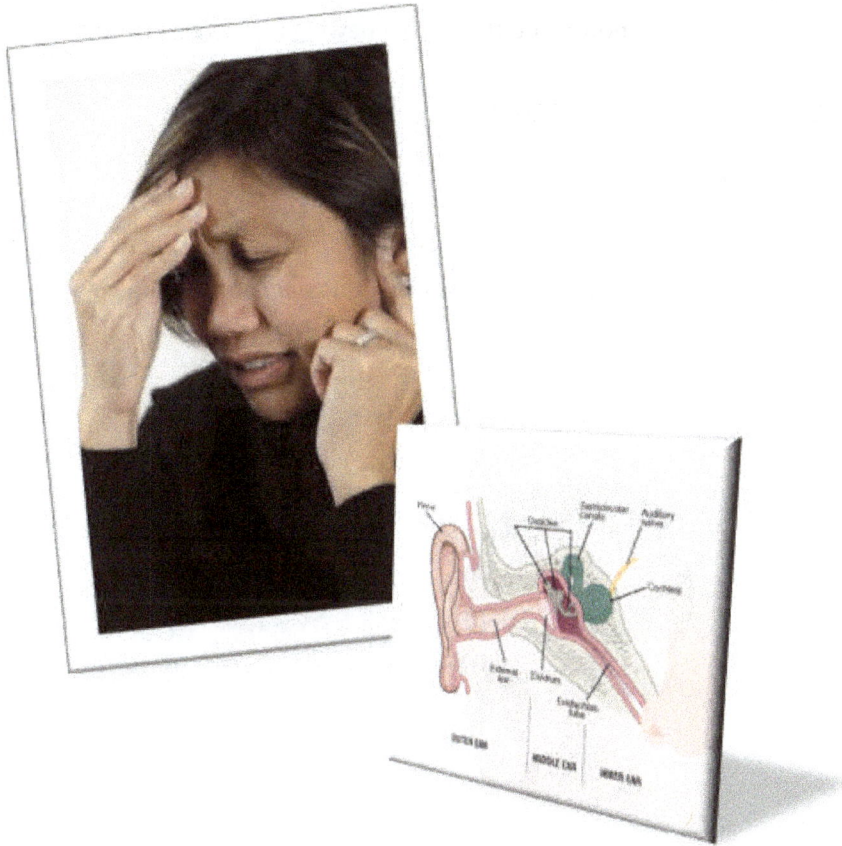

Pains in the ear, are most often, due to foreign body or insect entering the auditory canal. However, there are diseases which can cause pain in the ear that needs immediate attention. Some maybe trivial, but others, could be life threatening.

PAIN IN THE EAR + FULLNESS

Pain in the ear associated with the feeling of fullness and /or deafness aggravated by pulling the ear lobe on one side. Fever is sometimes noted and the act of chewing may aggravate the pain.

DIAGNOSIS: FURUNCLE OF THE AUDITORY CANAL

ORGAN INVOLVE: *auditory canal*

CAUSE:

There is an infection and formation of abscess inside the ear canal due to vigorous act of cleaning and usage of sharp instruments.

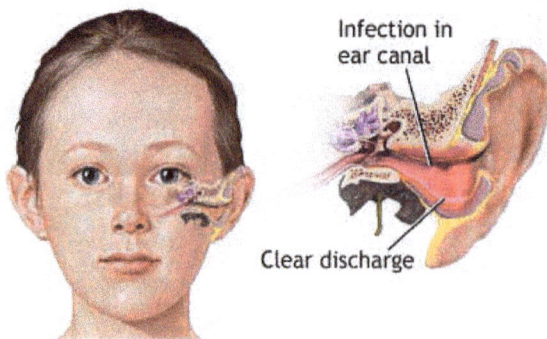

Infection in ear canal

Clear discharge

INITIAL TREATMENT:

    Adult: *GENTAMICIN EAR DROPS 2 drops 3x a day for 7 days*

    MEFENAMIC ACID 500 mg 1 tab every 4 hrs.
    CLOXACILLIN 500 mg 1 cap 3x a day for 7 days
    Children: CLOXACILLIN SYRUP 1 tsp. 3x a day for 7 days

ADVICE:

The use of sharp instruments in cleaning the ear is the common cause of infection. Done by barbers or any untrained personnel, ear cleaning is hazardous. Ear wax only occurs on the outer portion of the auditory canal and one does not need to poke the cleaning of the ear.

LABORATORY EXAMINATION: *none*

DEFINITIVE TREATMENT:

INCISION AND DRAINAGE – the drainage of the abscess is done by incising the mound with a stab knife.

PAIN IN THE EAR + ITCHINESS

Pain in the ear usually associated with severe itchiness aggravated by manipulating the ear. When cotton buds clean the ear, black particles could be extracted from the inside.

DIAGNOSIS: ACTINOMYCOSIS

ORGAN INVOLVE: external auditory canal

CAUSE: fungal infection

INITIAL TREATMENT: cotton buds soaked with hydrogen peroxide (Agua oxigenada)

ADVICE:

Most fungal infection of the ear comes from contaminated instruments used in the cleaning of the ear such as those used in barber shops and beauty parlor. Fungal infection of the ear is difficult to eradicate. Long standing infection can be completely cured with prolonged treatment with anti-fungal medications both oral and topical. Constant cleaning is the primary mode of treatment.

LABORATORY EXAMINATION:

KOH OF EAR DISCHARGE – is the best way to identify the fungus responsible.

ESOPHAGOGRAM – x-ray procedure whereby the patient is asked to swallow milky substance and x-ray is taken in the act swallowing. This may visualize stricture or mass inside the esophagus. Not diagnostic in terms of determining malignancy.

DEFINITIVE TREATMENT:

CANESTEN EAR DROPS 2 drops 4x a day.

Chapter Two

Reddening and Wounds

REDDENING AND WOUNDS

This chapter discusses some basic knowledge on reddening to enable the reader to clarify the nature of the disease and to understand the physician.

Reddening of any part in the body is an indication of active blood supply to the affected part due to infection, trauma, abnormal growth or malformation of blood vessels. This reaction is a physiologic protective mechanism of the body to preserve the affected part. In infection, this reaction is a containment mechanism of the body to prevent spread of the foreign invader. Likewise, in trauma, which is the start of the rebuilding mechanism whereby, the destroyed tissues are immediately repaired by the delivery of basic parts. In other instances, like abnormal growth of cancerous tumor, the reddening of the body part indicates massive blood supply to the abnormal tissue build up. It is often the pathognomonic sign of cancer that pathologist look for in diagnosis. Also, in blood vessel malformation, such as, ARTERIOVENOUS FISTULA, the reddening indicates abnormal formation of blood vessels concentrated in one location.

Thus, the information given in the following pages are intended for the reader to understand the mechanism of the reddening of the affected part (*RUBOR* - Latin word for reddening). Treatment follows the diagnosis to give the reader the inkling of what doctors usually follow in the management of the affected area. The reader is cautioned, however, that there are diseases which manifest as reddening, and yet, there is a much graver problem associated with it. And self-medication may complicate matters, like diseases affecting the eye. Therefore, consultation with a physician is the best step to do.

REDDENING AND DARK
DISCOLORATIONS OF THE SKIN

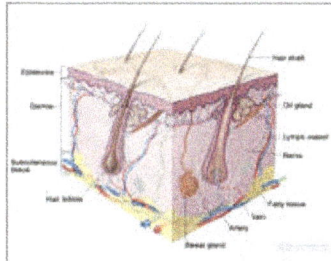

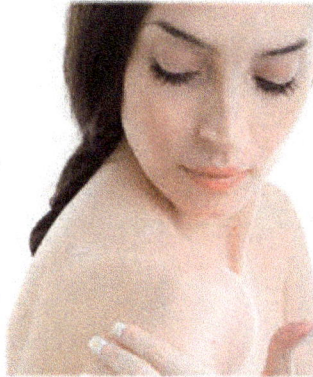

Reddening of the skin indicates infection and the formation of abscess. Some infections of the skin do not manifest as swelling but the spread of reddish area and marked demarcation of the normal skin from the abnormal is by its color. Tenderness usually compounds the problem and the affected area is warm.

Some systematic diseases manifest as reddening of the skin and should be dealt with by the reader in its entirety. Though far off, these accompanying symptoms should be searched throughout the body before making a diagnosis. The absence of the accompanying symptoms, however, does not exclude the possibility of illness. The sharpness of thought of the reader will be revealed, and most often, can mislead him or her to other conclusions, in the same way, that symptoms, cannot often be diagnosed by a doctor. When treatment involves radical steps, the reader should not proceed with the suggested therapy, unless, he fully understands the consequences. A discussion with his doctor should be undertaken prior to the signing of the consent in order to fully grasp the situation at hand.

REDDENING OF THE SKIN POST-TRAUMA

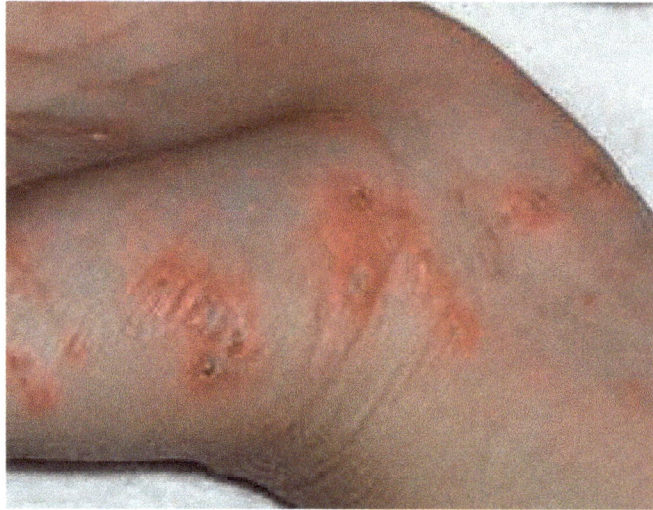

Reddening of the skin in any area of the body after trauma due to fall, vehicular accident, mauling or self-inflicted.

DIAGNOSIS: CONTUSION

ORGAN INVOLVED: *subcutaneous area of skin*

CAUSE: break of the underlying blood vessels due to trauma

INITIAL TREATMENT:

COLD COMPRESS - is used rather than warm. This stops further bleeding of the affected area and initiates coalition of the blood clot.

ADVICE:

Disappearance of the reddening cannot be accomplished in 24 hours. It usually takes 3 days. Taking of antibiotics is unnecessary. Analgesics may help but do not enhance immediate disappearance. Hemostatic and those medicines which promote blood clotting do not hasten healing and disappearance. Medicines such as Aspirin prevents blood clotting and do further damage by allowing further bleeding.

LABORATORY EXAMINITION:

X-RAYS - determines any damage to the underlying bones. Soft tissue damage cannot be visualized by this modality and is therefore not recommended to determine the existence of blood clot, nerve and muscle damage.

DEFINITIVE TREATMENT:

Treatment of the underlying damage such as bone fractures. Otherwise, NONE.

HEMATOMA

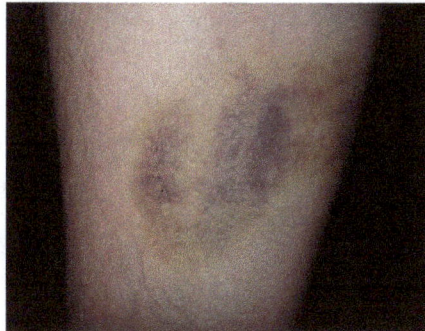

Reddening of the skin secondary trauma or mauling, which is usually followed by darkening of the area as blood clot expands.

DIAGNOSIS: HEMATOMA

ORGAN INVOLVED: subcutaneous blood vessels

CAUSE: breaking of underlying blood vessels under the skin

INITIAL TREAMENT: COLD COMPRESS - to stop the bleeding underneath the skin.
MEFENAMIC ACID 500 mg 1 tab every 4 hours for pain

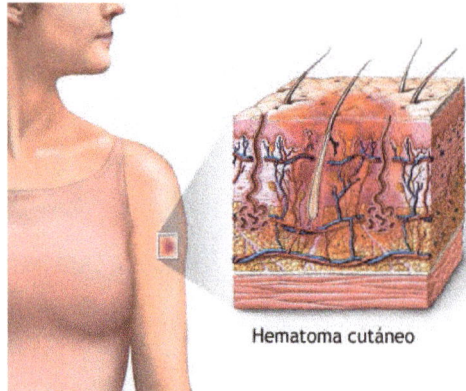

Hematoma cutáneo

ADVICE:

Antibiotics are not necessary in these cases most especially if there is no break in the skin or wound. Hematomas usually subside in 4 to 5 days and no medication can hasten healing. A yellowish discoloration of the area follows when the blood clot dissipates followed by disappearance of the entire lesion.

LABORATORY EXAMINITION:

X-RAY – determines the possibility of fractures of bones underneath the injury.

DEFINITIVE TREATMENT:

Treatment is directed towards accompanying injuries such as fractures.

INSECT BITE

Reddening and swelling of the skin due to insect bites which are not venomous.

DIAGNOSIS: ANGIOEDEMA SECOND

TO INSECT BITE

ORGAN INVOLVED: *skin*

CAUSE: Insect bite non venomous

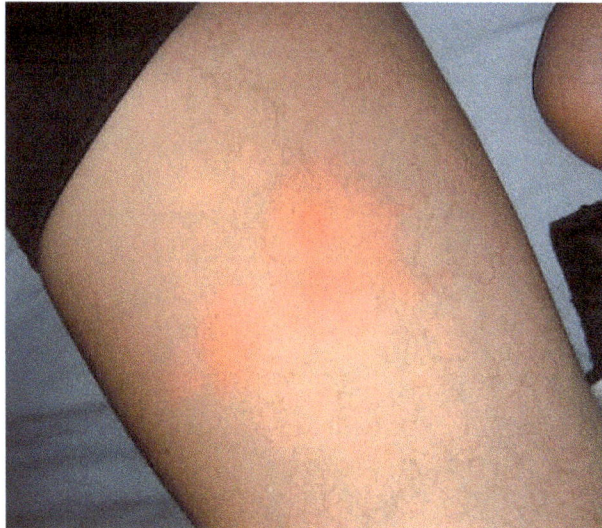

INITIAL TREATMENT:
    COLD COMPRESS on the affected area
    CITIRIZINE 1 tab daily for 5 days

ADVICE:

      Swelling of the skin secondary to insect bite that is not venomous can subside without treatment. Even with cold compress alone, the affected area may decrease in size and pain may be diminished. Some insect bites may cause systematic reaction such as rashes and swelling of the face. Some insect bites may cause death due to anaphylaxis: severe allergy causing difficulty of breathing.

LABORATORY EXAMINATION: *none*

DEFINITIVE TRAETMENT:

      For systemic severe allergy secondary to insect bite:

            CITIRIZINE INJECTION 1 amp im

            SOLU CORTEF 500 mg 1vial im

SKIN INFECTION

Reddening of the skin associated with pain and swelling and tenderness when touched. Some people develop fever and swelling of nearby lymph nodes.

DIAGNOSIS: ERYTHEMA

ORGAN INVOLVED: *skin*

CAUSE: staphylococcal infection of the skin

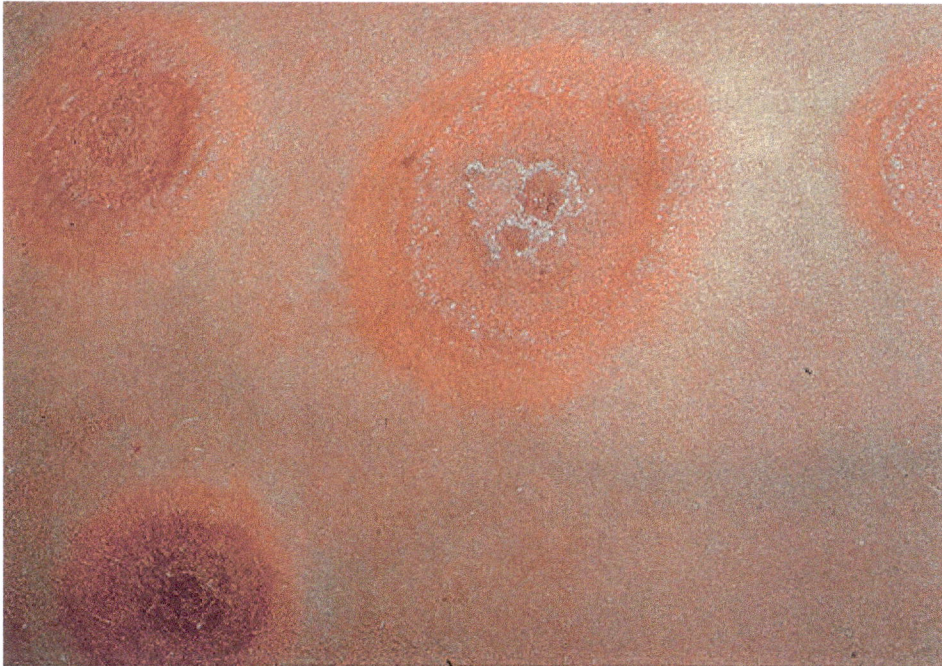

INITIAL TREATMENT:

ANALGESICS: MEFENAMIC ACID 500 mg tablet every 4 hrs for 3 days

ANTIBIOTICS: CLOXCILLIN 500 mg 1 cap 3x a day for 7 days

ADVICE:

Most swelling of the skin may subside with initial antibiotics. But some may continue to develop into an abscess (see Abscess). Complete treatment is necessary to prevent further treatment such as incision and drainage, which require surgery.

LABORATORY EXAMINATION: *none*

DEFINITIVE TREATMENT: *none*

ABSCESS

Reddening of the skin followed by formation of pus

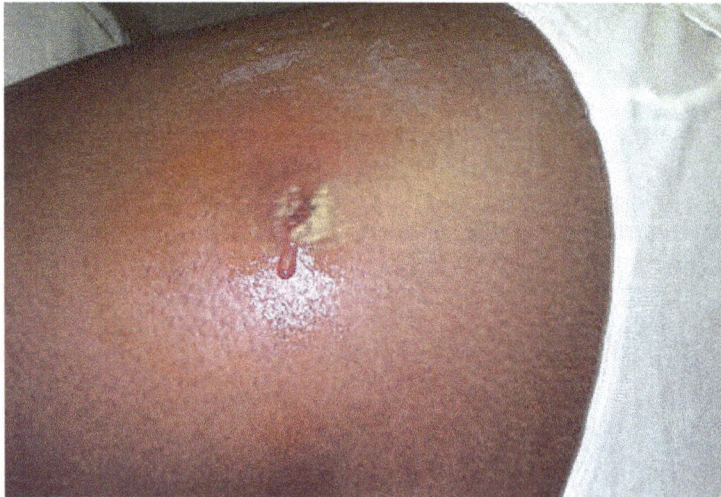

DIAGNOSIS: ABSCESS FORMATION

ORGAN INVOLVED: subcutaneous tissue

CAUSE: staphylococcus infection

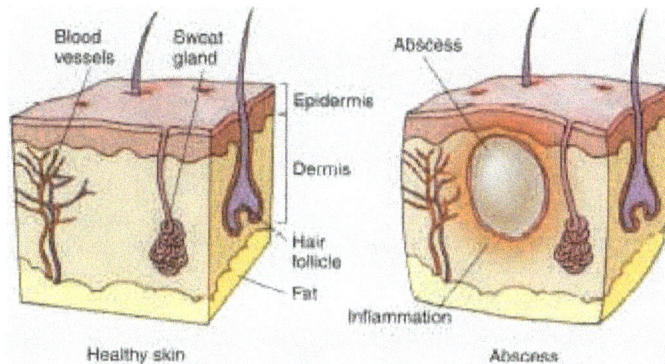

Healthy skin   Abscess

INITIAL TREATMENT:

    ANTIBIOTICS: CLOXACILLIN 500 mg 1 cap 3x a day for 7 days

    ANALGESICS: DICLOFENAC NA 50 mg tablet every 4 hours

ADVICE:

    Even with sufficient antibiotics, abscesses do not subside and heal because the pus persists inside the skin. Incision and drainage is necessary to remove the pus which prevents healing; the earlier the surgery, the faster the healing.

LABORATORY EXAMINATION:

    CULTURE AND SENSITIVITY – growing of pus in the lab to determine the presence of bacteria if the wound does not heal with ordinary antibiotics.

DEFINITIVE TREATMENT:

    INCISION AND DRAINAGE – draining out pus with a small lancet after local anesthesia. A small rubber drain is inserted to prevent premature closure of the wound. Dressing is necessary the next day to remove the rubber drain.

    ANTIBIOTICS:

PROSTAPHLIN 500 mg 1 cap 3x a day for 7 days

ANALGESICS:
MEFENAMIC ACID 500 mg 1 cap every 4 hours

FURUNCULOSIS

Multiple reddening and pus formation of the skin

DIAGNOSIS: FURUNCULOSIS

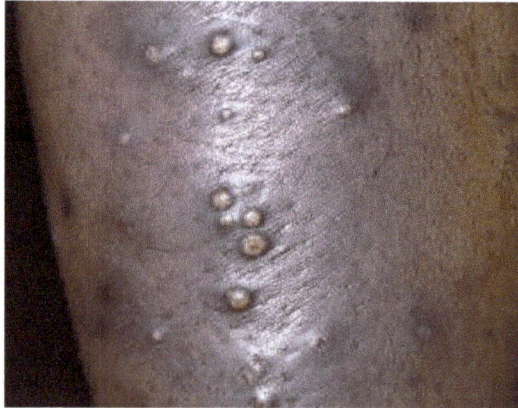

ORGAN INVOLVED: *skin*

CAUSE: staphylococcus infection of the skin

INITIAL TREATMENT:
>   WASH with soap and water 2x a day
>   GARAMYCIN OINTMENT – to be applied with dressing 2x a day
>   ANTIBIOTIC: PROSTAPHLIN 500 mg 1 cap 3x a day for 7 days

ADVICE:

Most infection like this occurs when the person has decreased immune system such as in AIDS. But they also occur in places where hygiene is not observed. If not treated, the infection may become serious and develop into ulceration or wound with exposure of the underlying muscle.

LABORATORY EXAMINATION:

Culture and sensitivity – to determine the bacteria causing the infection

DEFINITIVE TREATMENT:

DEBRIDEMENT – removal of the pus formations by sharp dissection after application of local anesthesia such as MLAC.

DRESSING – application of wound ointments embedded on dressings such as SILVER SULFADIAZINE
ANTIBIOTICS: PROSTAPHLIN 500 mg 4x a day for 1 week.

INFECTED SEBACEOUS CYST

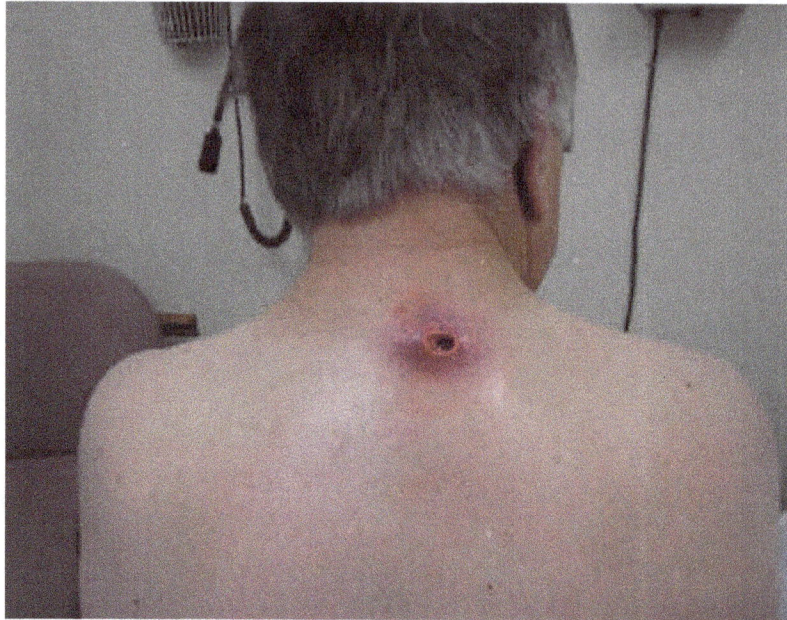

Reddening
formerly innocuous
tender, fluctuant

of a mass
which become
and painful on palpation

DIAGNOSIS: INFECTED SEBACEOUS CYST

ORGAN INVOLVED: skin cyst formation

CAUSE: staphylococcal infection of the cyst

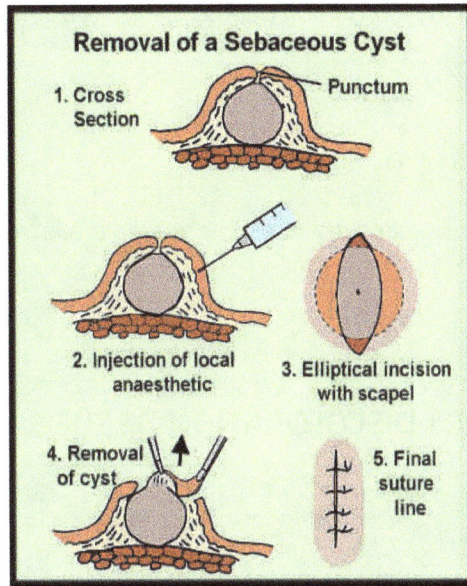

Removal of a Sebaceous Cyst

1. Cross Section — Punctum
2. Injection of local anaesthetic
3. Elliptical incision with scapel
4. Removal of cyst
5. Final suture line

INITIAL TREATMENT:

ANTIBIOTIC:

CLOXACILLIN 500 mg 1 cap 3x a day for 7 days

ANALGESIC:

MEFENAMIC ACID 500 mg 1 cap every 4 hours

ADVICE:

Sebaceous cysts are inclusion cyst that starts from hair follicles which when plugged by dirt and grime, they enlarge and form into a cyst. More often than not, because of the content of these cysts, they become infected and develop into an abscess. When the cyst is discovered, excision is a must rather than waiting for it to enlarge or get infected.

LABORATORY EXAMINATION: *NONE*

DEFINITIVE TREATMENT:

INCISION AND DRAINAGE – the evacuation of pus by making a small incision on top of the abscess after infiltration of local anesthesia.

ANTIBIOTIC
CLOXACILLIN 500 mg 1cap 3x a day for 7 days

TOTAL EXCISION – After incision and drainage, the wound is allowed to heal. Total excision is done when the cyst reappears.

DARK DISCOLORATION OF THE SKIN

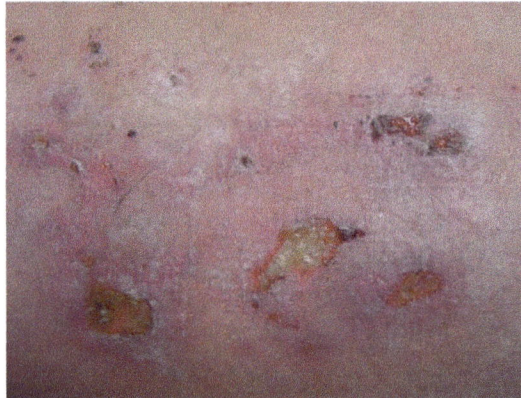

Dark patches of the skin that become systemic and cover the whole body. They are usually non-itchy and painless.

DIAGNOSIS: EXCORIATIONS

ORGAN INVOLVED: subcutaneous blood vessels

CAUSE: leukemia, uremia, liver failure and other blood related diseases like diabetes

INITIAL TREATMENT: *none*

ADVICE:

This is a manifestation of a grave illness that needs immediate medical consultation. There are other hosts of diseases that manifest by these skin findings. Thorough laboratory examination is the only way to determine diagnosis.

LABORATORY EXAMINATION:

PERIPHERAL SMEAR – to determine blood dyscrasias and other blood related diseases like leukemia, anemia.

CREATININE – blood examination to determine the function of the kidney. Kidney failure may manifest as skin excoriations.

SGPT-SGOT (ALT) – to determine liver function. Liver failure may also manifest as skin excoriations.

FASTING BLOOD SUGAR - determines the presence of diabetes

DEFINITIVE TREATMENT:

KIDNEY DIALYSIS – for kidney failure

CHEMOTHERAPY - for leukemia and other blood related illnesses

LIVER TRANSPLANT – for liver failure

CAT BITE

Reddening of the skin due to a house cat bite

DIAGNOSIS: PUNCTURED WOUND

ORGAN INVOLVED: *skin*

CAUSE: cat bite

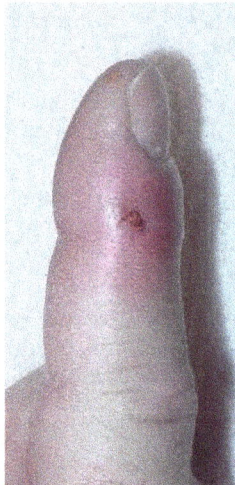

INITIAL TREATMENT: Wash with soap and water
    ANTIBIOTIC:
        Adult: PROSTAPHLIN 250 mg 1 cap 3x a day for 7 days
        Children: PROSTAPHLIN SYRUP 1 tsp. 4x a day for 7 days

    ANALGESIC:
        Adult: MEFENAMIC ACID 250 mg tablet every 4 hours
        Children: MEFENAMIC SYRUP 1 tsp every 4 hours

ADVICE: House cats do not carry rabies. Cat bites cause infection and tetanus.

DEFINITIVE TREATMENT:

HUMAN ANTI-TETANUS IMMUNE *GLOBULIN* 250 *uim* – for immediate coverage against tetanus if patient has never been given tetanus vaccination in the past or for the last ten years. This injection only last for 30 days.

TETANUS TOXOID 1 AMP IM – for tetanus coverage 30 days after bite and the only one given for patients who have complete vaccination prior to the bite. This will serve as a booster dose.

ANTIBIOTIC: PROSTAPHLIN 250 mg 1 cap 3x a day for 7 days

DOG BITE

Punctured wound or laceration after dog bite

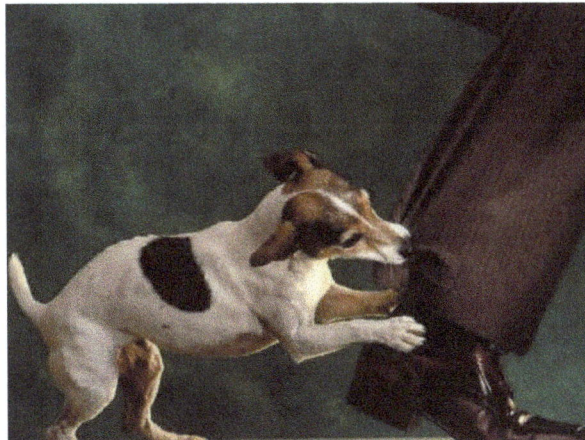

DIAGNOSIS: Punctured Wound or Laceration Secondary to Dog Bite

ORGAN INVOLVED:

Location of the dog bite is important. Above the shoulder bite needs immediate injection of anti-RABIES immune globulin. Below the shoulder, an anti-rabies vaccine may be used.

INITIAL TREATMENT:

Wash the affected area with soap and water. Keep open unless bleeding.

ADVICE:

Preservation of the dog's life is very important to determine if it is rabid or not. But if possible, the dog's head must be brought to the laboratory for examination of the brain for presence of rabies. Any other treatment outside of anti-rabies injection does not protect the patient from rabies.

DEFINITIVE TREATMENT:

ANTI-RABIES HUMAN IMMUNOGLOBULIN 300 U IM

- to be given if the bite is above the shoulder; dog is determined to be rabid; or the dog cannot be found

ANTI-RABIES VACCINATION (VERORAB) IM

– Five injections given in specific days (1-3-7-14-21st day post bite)

ANTI-TETANUS HUMAN IMMUNOGLOBULIN 250 U IM

- dog bites also cause tetanus. Given if the patient does not have any tetanus vaccination in the past

ANTI-TETANUS VACCINATION 1 amp IM – for protection 30 days post bite.

INSECT BITE

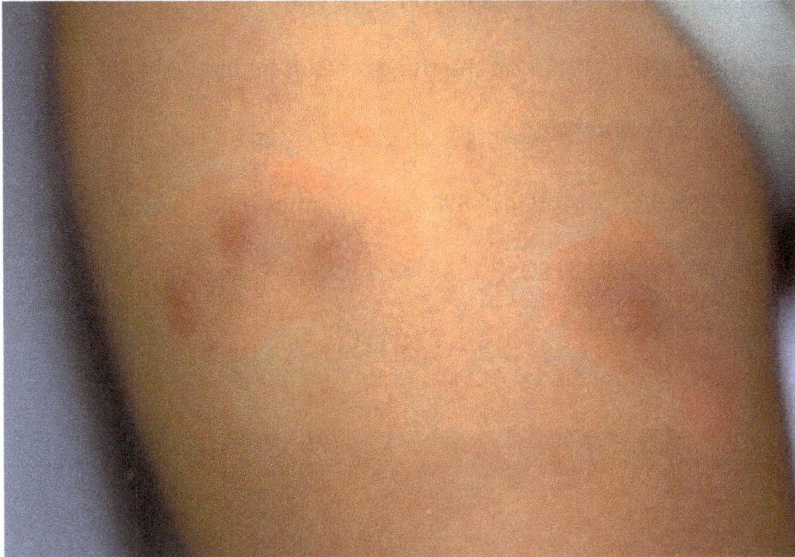

(Cockroach, Centipede, Bee Stings,)

Reddening of the skin associated with swelling and papule formation secondary to insect bite.

DIAGNOSIS: ERYTHEMA SECONDARY TO INSECT BITE

INITIAL TREATMENT:

COLD COMPRESS – to diminish the swelling and pain

WASH with soap and water – to diminish the histaminic effect of the insect bite

ADVICE:

If not treated, insect bites may lead to infection and wound ulceration. The objective of the treatment is to neutralize any venomous effect of the insect bite. Some bites may lead to anaphylaxis (severe allergic reaction) causing difficulty of breathing and subsequent death. If the patient has a history of severe reaction to insect bites, patient must be brought to the hospital for proper definitive treatment.

LABORATORY EXAMINATION: *none*

DEFINITIVE TREATMENT:

ADULT: ANTIHISTAMINES – CETIRIZINE tablet once a day for 5 days

ANTIHISTAMINE INJECTION – on the site of the insect bite

ANTIBIOTIC: AMOXYCILLIN 500 mg 1 cap 3x a day for 5 days

CHILDREN: ANTIHISTAMINES - CETIRIZINE SYRUP 1 tsp. once daily

ANTIBIOTIC: AMOXYCILLIN SUSP 1 tsp. 4x a day for 7 days

RAT BITE

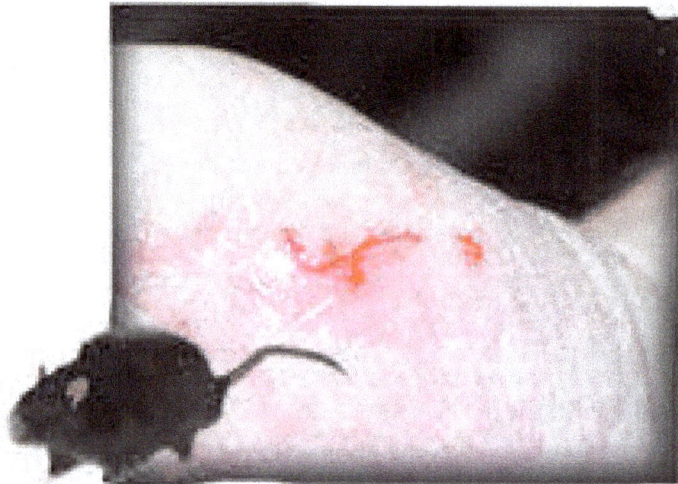

Reddening of the skin secondary to rat bite

DIAGNOSIS: PUNCTURED WOUND

INITIAL TREATMENT: WASH with soap and water

ADVICE:

City rats do not carry rabies. Only wild rats due to its association with wild animals get infected with rabies. Tetanus and severe infection are the main problems with rat bites. They progress into massive wound ulcerations if not given the right antibiotics. Some rat bites need debridement and cleaning. Inflammation of lymph nodes and fever indicates severe infection. Systemic infection has been known to arise from rat bites including RAT BITE SPOTTED FEVER. In these instances, admission of the patient to the hospital is necessary.

LABORATORY EXAMINATION:

COMPLETE BLOOD COUNT - to determine presence of systemic infection

DEFINITIVE TREATMENT:

TETANUS HUMAN IMMUNOGLOBULIN 250 u IM – to all patientswith no immunization

TETANUS TOXOID VACCINE 1 amp IM – to all patients with no immunization and with immunization of more than 5 years

ANTIBIOTICS: PROSTAPHLIN 500 mg 1 cap 3x a day for 7 days

CHILDREN: ANTIBIOTIC PROSTAPHLIN SUSP 1 tsp. 3x a day for 1 week

HUMAN BITE

Wounds or lacerations sustained after a human bite

DIAGNOSIS: LACERATIONS SECONDARY TO HUMAN BITE

INITIAL TREATMENT:

WASH with soap and water. Control bleeding by putting pressure on top of the wound with clean cloth.

ANTIBIOTICS: PROSTAPHLIN 500 mg 1 cap 3x aday for 7 days

ANALGESICS: MEFENAMIC ACID 500 mg tablet every 4 hours

ADVICE:

Human bite does not carry rabies or tetanus. Infection is more likely due to bacteria in the mouth. Washing with soap and water diminish the infection. What's important is to approximate the lacerated wound for cosmetic and psychological result. For medico-legal purposes, the size, depth and shape of the wound should be measured; time and location of affliction. A medical certificate issued by the physician is more important than the treatment.

LABORATORY EXAMINATION: *none*

DEFENITIVE TREATMENT:

SUTURING OF THE WOUND – wounds if they are more than 2 cm should be sutured back for cosmetic as well as legal purposes.

ANTIBIOTIC: PROSTAPHLIN 500 mg 1 cap 3x a day for 7 days

SUPERFICIAL WOUNDS

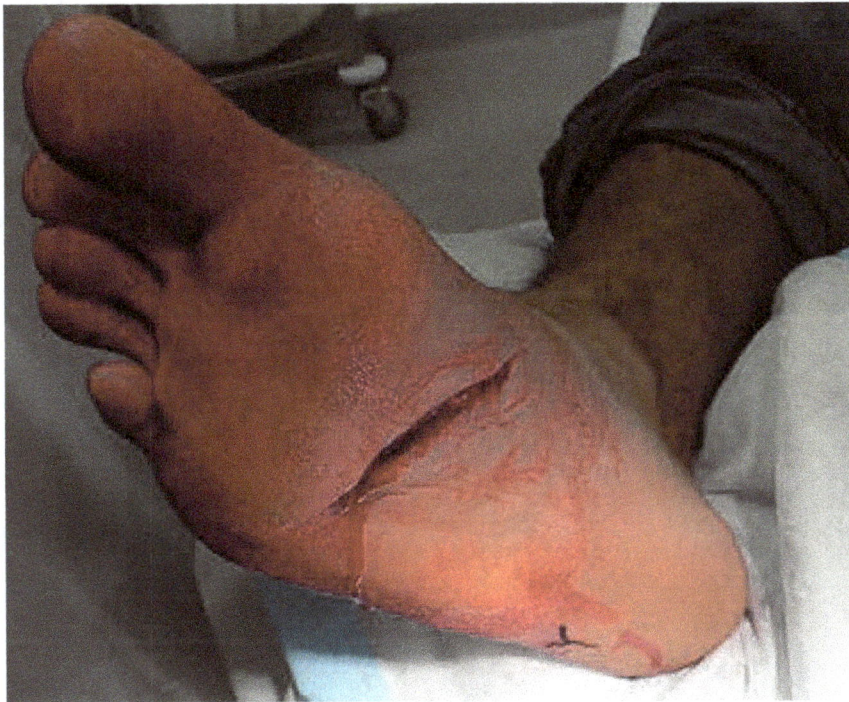

(Nail, barbecue stick, glass, metal, knife)

Superficial wounds sustained in the foot, hand, arm, and scalp but not in the chest, abdomen, neck or face.

DIAGNOSIS: If depth could not be determined, immediate consultation with a physician is necessary.

ORGAN INVOLVED: Wounds sustained in the chest and abdomen is difficult to measure. Laboratory examinations are necessary.

INITIAL TREATMENT:

Wash with soap and water - grime and dirt should be removed immediately to minimize infection. Pressure on top of the wound will check bleeding. *Betadine, alcohol or iodine are not necessary for cleaning. They delay wound healing.*

ADVICE:

Immediate cleaning of the wound diminishes infection. Soap and water is the right solution and no other. If the offending nail or glass is stuck in the wound, do not attempt to remove. Bring patient to the hospital for the proper removal. Massive bleeding may ensue if these are removed improperly.

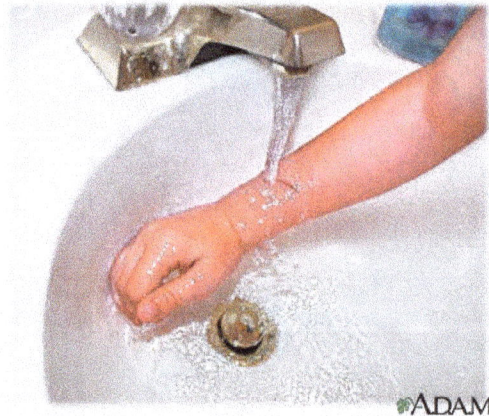

LABORATORY EXAMINATION:

X-RAY OF THE AFFECTED area – foreign bodies may be left inside the wound. Thongs like glass may be missed even in good hands. Claims of the patient should be taken face value until otherwise proven wrong.

DEFINITIVE TREATMENT:

DEBRIDEMENT AND SUTURING – if the wound is more than 2 cm, suturing should be done to approximate the edges. They heal faster and complications are lesser.

TETANUS HUMAN IMMUNOGLOBULIN 250 U IM – for those who have no immunization in the past.

TETANUS TOXOID VACCINE – for those who have no immunization or immunization was done more than 5 years ago.

ANTIBIOTICS: PROSTAPHLIN 500 mg 1 cap 3x a day for 7 days

SKIN ABSCESS WITHOUT OPENING

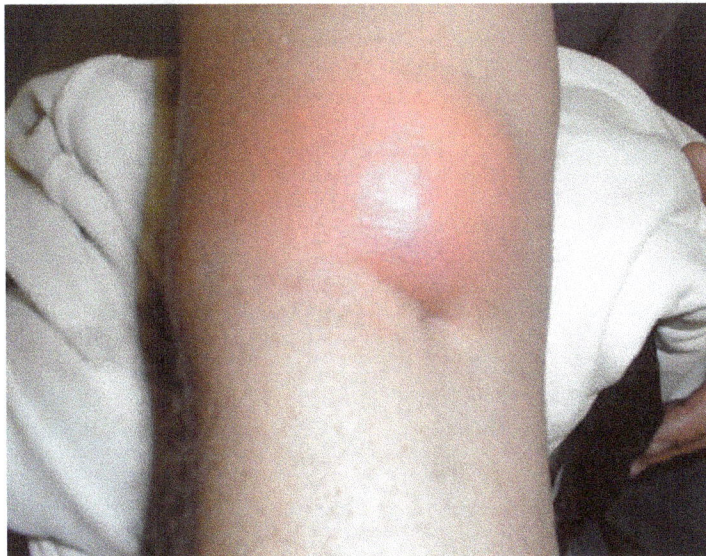

Abscess formation of the skin usually found in the buttocks and armpit

DIAGNOSIS: SKIN ABSCESS

CAUSE: STAPHYLOCOCCAL INFECTION OF THE SKIN

INITIAL TREATMENT:
        CLOXACILLIN 500 mg 1 cap 3x a day for 7 days
        MEFENAMIC ACID 500 mg tablet every 4 hrs for pain

ADVICE: Skin abscess left alone without surgery even with antibiotic intake will heal longer than necessary. Pus formation inside the abscess prevents tissue healing thereby prolonging pain. Surgery hastens healing.

LABORATORY EXAMINATION: not necessary

DEFINITIVE TREATMENT:

INCISION AND DRANAIGE – a small incision is made on top of the abscess to drain the pus. If it is not done, healing will take longer than usual 7 days.

PROSTAPHLIN (Cloxacillin sodium) 500 mg 1 cap 3x a day for 7 days

MEFENAMIC ACID 500 mg tablet every 4 hrs for pain

SKIN ABSCESS WITH PUSTULE

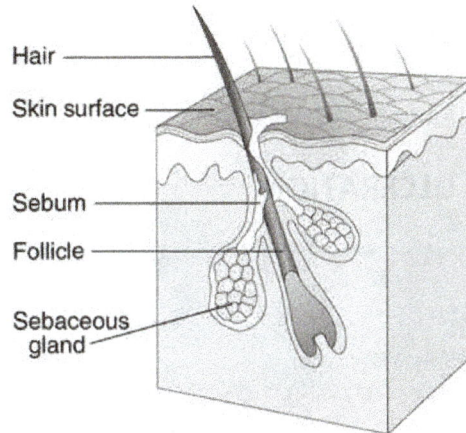
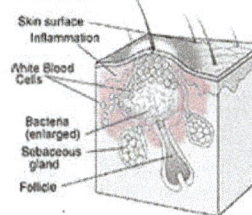

Abscess formation of the skin with pustule formation on top.

DIAGNOSIS: BREAKING SKIN ABSCESS

CAUSE: Skin on top of the abscess has necrosis leaving a yellowish spot made up of hard pus.

ADVICE: Hard pustule on top of an abscess plugs the exit of the pus forming under it. It is similar to an abscess without opening unless the pustule is removed.

LABORATORY EXAMINATION: not necessary

DEFINITIVE TREATMENT:
1. Removal of the hard pustule on top- It is necessary to remove this plug. This can be accomplished even without anesthesia by slowly picking the yellowish spot until it liquefies.
2. Further cleaning is done by introducing HYDROGEN PEROXIDE inside the abscess with the use of cotton buds. This may be painful but injection of anesthesia does not provide a painless procedure due to the acidity of the wound.

3. Administration of an ointment (GARAMYCIN OINTMENT) inside the abscess prevents further pus information in the future.
4. Dressing should be light in order for the pus to drain.

ANTIBIOTICS: Clindamycin–C 300 mg 1 cap 3x a day for 7 days

SKIN ULCERATION

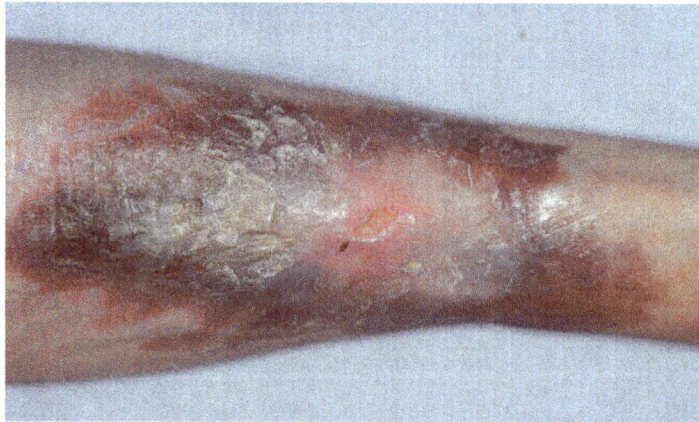

Large wound ulceration of the skin from an abscess that was not treated properly.

DIAGNOSIS: *WOUND ULCER*

CAUSE: Skin abscess, which have been left without treatment.

LABORATORY EXAMINATION:

FASTING BLOOD SUGAR – use to determine any presence of DIABETES MELLITUS. Most patients who develop this kind of abscess have diabetes.

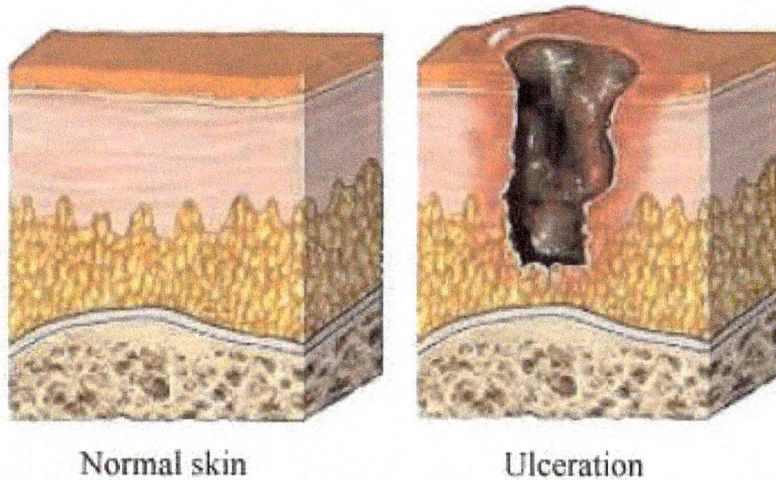

Normal skin   Ulceration

ADVICE:

Skin ulcerations are the result of abscess formation left alone without treatment. Necrosis has set inside the skin breaking into thin layer of pus. This exposes the underlying tissues such as the muscle and fascia and sometimes the bone. Wound healing will take 3 to 4 weeks and sometimes may need skin grafting from other locations of the body.

DEFINITIVE TREATMENT:

CEFUROXIME 500 mg tablet 3x a day for 10 days

DRESSING – Dressings should not be done daily in the following manner:

1. All dead tissues and pus formations should be removed inside the wound. This may necessitate cutting tissues (debridement).
2. Cleaning with hydrogen peroxide especially under cliff of the wound.
3. Impregnate FLAMMAZINE cream into pieces of gauze bandage and apply on the wound.
4. Add another layer of bandage on top. Do not apply any solution like betadine or anything over the wound. This will slow down proper healing.

WOUNDS AND BLUNT INJURY TO THE CHEST

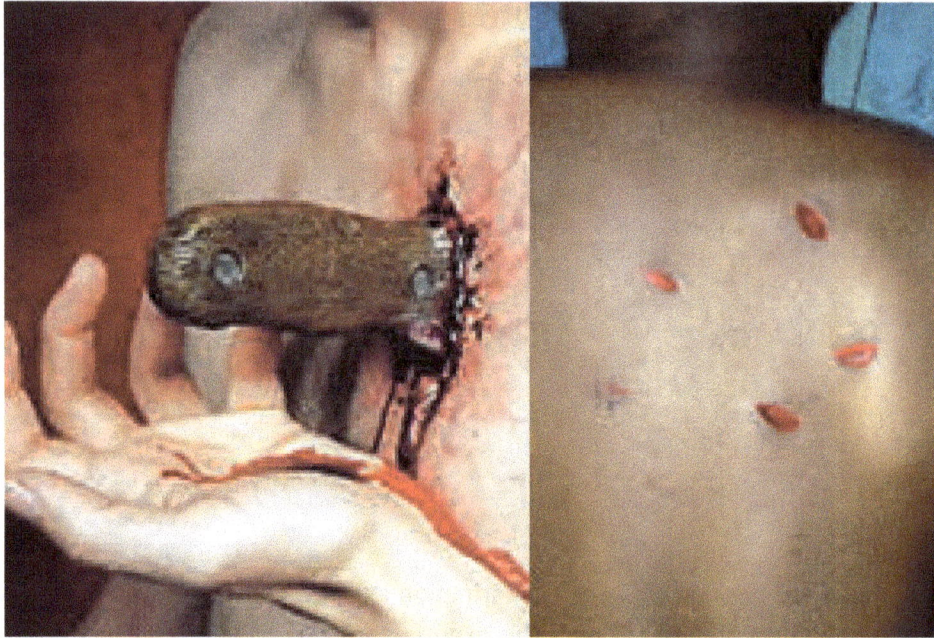

(Stabbed Wound, Gunshot Wound, Vehicular Accident)

Wounds of the chest sustained by stabbed wound, gunshot wound or in vehicular accidents whether they seemed to be superficial or deep.

DIAGNOSIS: PENETRATING OR NON-PENETRATING TO THE CHEST CAVITY

INITIAL TREATMENT:

CLOSURE OF THE WOUND - by any means to prevent suction of air into the chest cavity (i.e. cloth plug)

ADVICE:

Difficulty of breathing is one indication that the wound has penetrated the chest cavity. In the absence of this, there is no assurance that the inflicted wound is superficial. Only diagnostic x-rays could determine this. Probing of the wound by any means outside or inside the hospital does not make a diagnosis. It may worsen a superficial wound and convert it into a penetrating wound. If patient is asymptomatic and Chest x-rays show negative findings, admission is necessary for observation. Bullets inside the chest cavity in patients who do not have any symptoms do not need extraction or surgery. They are better left alone than doing surgery to remove.

LABORATORY EXAMINATION:

CHEST X-RAY - Stabbed wounds when it has penetrated the chest cavity, no matter how small the entry wound is, will show as ATELECTASIS (collapse of the lungs) or HEMOTHORAX (blood in the lungs)
- Gunshot wounds may pass through the chest cavity to the other side of the body without inflicting any harm to the lung parenchyma. But most often may produce HEMOTHORAX (blood in the chest cavity) AND PNEUMOTHORAX (air in the chest cavity) with subsequent ATELECTASIS.
- Fractures of the ribs necessitate stabilization.

DEFINITIVE TREATMENT: *ADMISSION TO THE HOSPITAL*

CHEST TUBE INSERTION (THORACOSTOMY) - opening on the side of the chest and insertion of a tube into the chest cavity for drainage of HEMOTHORAX AND PNEUMOTHORAX. The chest tube is attached to a bottle filled with 2 inches of water where the other end of the tube is immersed to prevent air from entering into the lungs during inspiration but allow air to escape from the lungs in expiration.

ANTIBIOTICS: PEN-G-NA 2 MILLION U EVERY 6 HRS IVTT ANST

TETANUS HUMAN IMMUNOGLOBULIN 250 UIM

TETANUS TOXOID VACCINE

ANLAGESICS: MEFENAMIC ACID 500 mg tablet every 4hrs

STABILIZATION OF RIB FRACTURES – if rib fracture is single, mere application of wide plaster is the only treatment. But if rib fractures are multiple and are causing flail of the rib cage, stabilization with the use of towel clips practically hanging the patient or the use of ventilators have to be resorted to.

WOUNDS AND BLUNT INJURY TO THE ABDOMEN

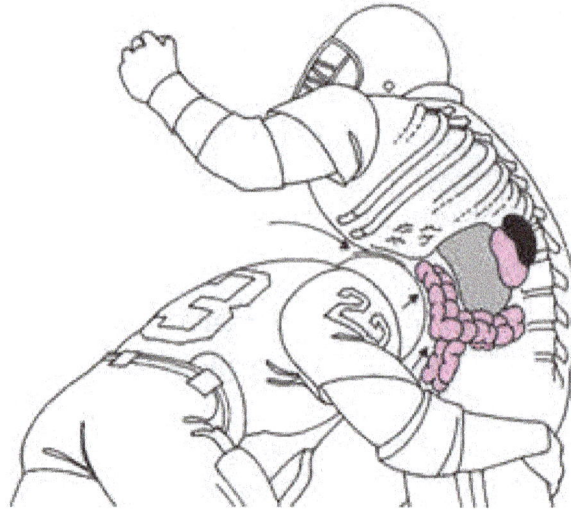

(Stabbed Wound, Gunshot Wound, Vehicular Accident)

Wounds in the abdomen sustained by sharp instruments, bullets and blunt injuries such as in vehicular accidents

DIAGNOSIS: Rest on whether it is penetrating or non-penetrating to the abdominal cavity.

INITIAL TREATMENT:

COVER on the wound to prevent evisceration (or coming out) of intestines and hemorrhage

ADVICE:

Treatment of injuries to the abdomen rests on the factor on whether the injury is penetrating or non-penetrating. In both instances, however, the patient has to be brought to the hospital to determine other related injuries which could be ascertained only thru diagnostic work-up. Probing of the wound in the hospital setting may be helpful in the diagnosis.

LABORATORY EXAMINATIONS:

UPRIGHT FILM OF THE ABDOMEN – an x- ray procedure taken with the patient standing up or sitting down a position that allows air that penetrated into the abdominal cavity to rest below the diaphragm. This is indicative of wound penetration.

PERITONEAL LAVAGE – A small incision is made below the navel under local anesthesia. A tube is inserted through the wound and several liters of dextrose water are poured into the abdomen through this tube. After several minutes, the water is suctioned back and examined for traces of blood and feces the presence of which indicate injury of the intestines and abdominal organs.

CT SCAN OF THE ABDOMINAL CAVITY – hemorrhage and pooling of blood in the abdomen can be detected by this procedure. Any injury to the liver and spleen no matter how small it is can be seen by this exam.

ULTRASOUND OF THE LIVER AND SPLEEN – the fastest way to diagnose any injury to the liver or spleen.

DEFINITIVE TREATMENT:

EXPLORATORY LAPAROTOMY – upon confirmation of penetration, the patient is brought to the OPERATING ROOM. Under GENERAL ANESTHESIA, an incision is made on his abdomen from the uppermost portion down to the lowest portion of the abdomen below the umbilicus. A complete examination of the entire abdomen including all parts of the intestines, liver, spleen, kidneys, colon and stomach is done. Injuries to these organs sustained not more than 4 hours are immediately closed. If this golden hour is breached (more than 5 hours since injury), the colon is exteriorized and brought out on another wound for future closure. Primary closure of these intestinal segments at this time invites disaster since they usually dehisced (reopen).

TETANUS HUMAN IMMUNOGLOBULIN 250 U IM
TETANUS TOXOID VACCINE 1 amp IM
ANTIBIOTICS: PEN-G-NA 2M units every 6 hours IVTTANST
ANALGESICS: NUBAIN 1 amp every 8 hours IVTT

WOUNDS AND BLUNT INJURYTO THE NECK

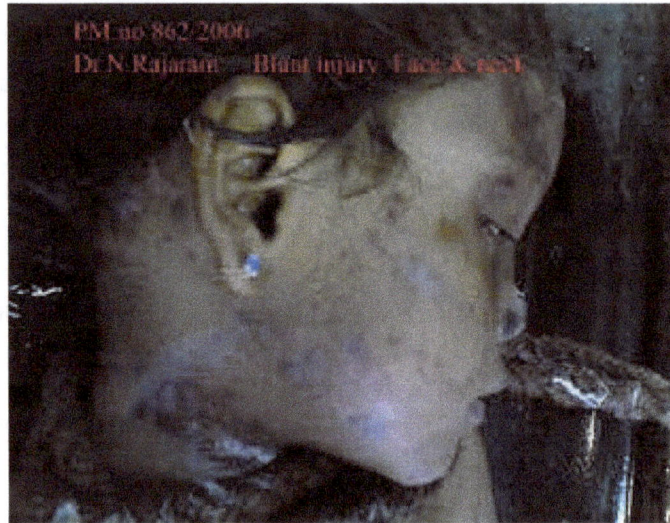

Wounds sustained in the neck whether by a knife, ice pick, or blunt trauma as in whiplash (car accidents) injuries, fall or mauling.

DIAGNOSIS: INJURY TO THE NECK BLOOD VESSELS, SOFT TISSUES AND NECK BONES

INITIAL TREATMENT:

BLEEDING should be allowed to flow freely rather than obstructing flow. Bleeding inside the neck causes breathing obstruction leading to asphyxia and death. Light dressings should be placed in front of the wound and not plugging it. If the accompanying persons know the location of the blood vessels involved, pressure should be applied on the source of the bleeding. If they do not, pressure should be applied on the wound.

BLUNT injuries to the neck usually cause fracture of the bones of the neck and the avulsion of the airways. Stabilization of the vertebral injury and cleaning the airway of debris (blood clots and dentures) are the most important initial procedure to be done. Placing the patient on his back face up and fixing his head with blocks heavy enough to prevent his head from turning is the next step to be done in order to stabilize the fracture.

ADVICE:

Sharp injuries to the neck have to be ascertained whether it is penetrating or not. In the presence of massive bleeding, the dilemma of whether to bring the patient to the hospital or not can easily be resolved. But in small wounds, which have clotted, this dilemma is very important to determine whether the patient could be sent home or the wound has to be explored. Injuries to the big blood vessels of the neck may present as small wounds but deep inside, a small clot is just holding a massive laceration. Exploration of these small wounds in the hospital is mandated to prevent catastrophe.

Blunt injuries to the neck present another problem in the resuscitation of the patient. Fractures of the cervical bone and trachea are the main cause of airway obstruction. Stabilization of these structures may save the patient.

LABORATORY EXAMINATION:

X-RAY OF THE NECK – presence of air in the subcutaneous tissue indicates penetration but does not pinpoint the injured structure.

CT SCAN OF THE NECK – the best diagnostic tool to look for blood vessel injuries.

DEFINITIVE TREATMENT:

EXPLORATION OF THE NECK WOUND – under general anesthesia, the wound is widened and the big blood vessels of the neck are examined for possible injury. Immediate closures of these wounds are done with the use of vascular sutures. Injuries to the bronchial structures may not need further treatment unless they are causing difficulty of breathing to the patient. When it is causing difficulty of breathing, a temporary TRACHEOSTOMY is done. TRACHEOSTOMY is an emergency procedure wherein a wound is made below the Adam's apple and the windpipe (bronchus) is exposed. An opening is made on the bronchus itself and tracheostomy tube (a curve metal tube) is inserted to serve as an airway inlet-outlet. This procedure is difficult to do without proper instruments and lighting and should never be attempted outside of the hospital setting.

TETANUS HUMAN IMMUNOGLOBULIN 250U IM

TETANUS TOXOID VACCINE 1 amp IM

ANTIBIOTICS: PROSTAPHLIN 500 mg 1 cap 3x a day for 7 days

If patient can take oral medications

ANALGESICS: MEFENAMIC ACID 500 mg 1 cap every 4 hours

WOUNDS OF THE FACE

EYEBROW – Eyebrows should not be shaved. Suturing should be done with the eyebrows and approximation should be accurate. Debridement is not necessary. Steri-strips could be used in approximating wounds that are not oozing or bleeding. They are cosmetically better.

EYELIDS – In closure of the horizontal lacerations, care should be taken not to cause inversion of the eyelids. Vertical lacerations should be closed approximating the exact side to the other and parallel. Dressing is not necessary.

NASAL BRIDGE – if it is not gaping, do not suture. Steri-strips do a better job of approximation.

UPPER LIP – Hemostasis is important (no bleeding). Approximations must be accurate. Small fine sutures must be used. Suturing of the under muscles should be done prior to the closure of the buccal mucosa laceration (if there is any). Alignment of the skin edges is the dictum with small bite sutures.

CHEEK – the dilemma of surgeons is how to repair a laceration that is cosmetically accepted postoperatively. If they follow the LANGER'S line, the scar result is better.

POST INJURY MANAGEMENT:
    TETANUS HUMAN IMMUNOGLOBULIN 250 U IM
    TETANUS TOXOID VACCINE
    PROSTAPHLIN 500 mg 1 cap 4x a day for 5 days
    CONTRACTUBEX OINTMENT – may diminish scarring but has to be used for years.

BLOOD IN URINE

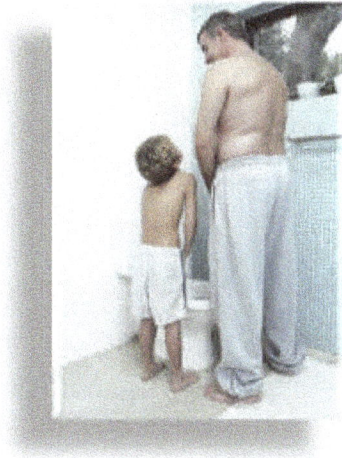

Reddening of the urine is caused by several factors. These factors are based on the URINARY TRACT section affected by disease. The URINARY TRACT is divided into KIDNEY, URETER, URINARY BLADDER, URETHRA and PROSTATE in the male. The accompanying symptoms usually indicate the level of the illness. In most cases, blood in the urine cannot be seen by the naked eye. Microscopic examination of the urine is necessary for detection of minute bleeding. Flank pains, as well as, pains located at the back and the abdomen usually indicate diseases of the kidneys and ureters. Hypogastric pains usually indicate diseases of the urinary bladder and prostate in the male. Pains radiating to the scrotum in the male (labia in the female) usually indicate stones impinging on the urinary bladder neck and lower third of the ureter. Some people develop numbness on the inner side of the thigh when stones are present in the ureter. These pains, accompanied by the presence of blood in the urine usually make diagnosis of urinary tract infection or stones in the urinary tract (URETEROLITHIASIS - stone in the ureter; CYSTOLITHIASIS - stone in the urinary bladder).

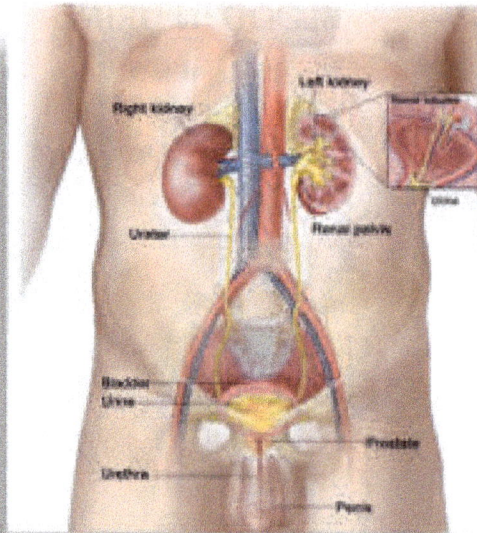

In the following pages, the reader is led to several diagnosis based on the presence of blood in the urine. This is presumed that blood could be seen in the urine or a urinalysis was done that showed RBC (RED BLOOD CELLS) in the urine.

BLOOD IN THE URINE + PAIN IN THE FLANKS

Blood urine associated with neither pain in the flanks with no fever nor pain during urination.

DIAGNOSIS: KIDNEY STONE

ORGAN INVOLVED: kidneys

CAUSE: stone formation

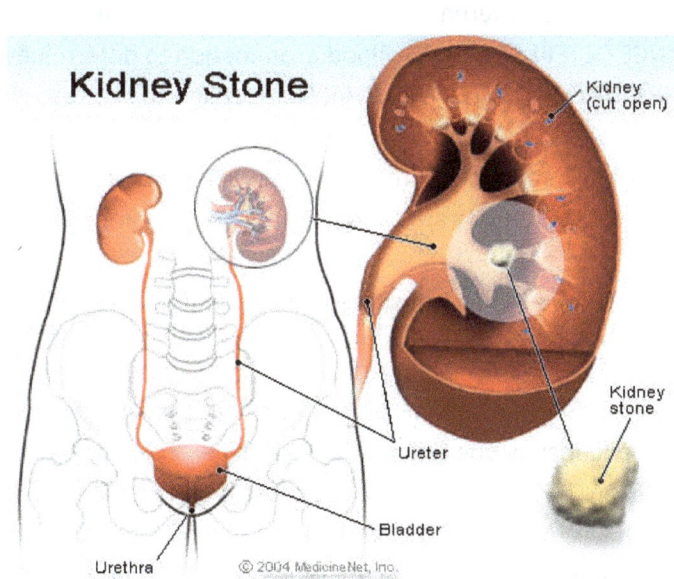

INITIAL TREATMENT:

    BUSCOPAN (Hyoscine butylbromide) 1 tab every 4 hrs. for pain

    BUCO JUICE 1 glass daily

    ACALKA (Potassium citrate) 1 tab 3x a day

    SAMBONG 1 tab 3x a day

ADVICE:

    Kidney stones are usually asymptomatic and do not cause pain. But when they start to descend down the ureter (the tube connecting the kidney and the urinary bladder), pain is felt whatever side is involved. The pain is characterized as heavy and piercing and most often involved the flanks of the abdomen. When kidney stones block the flow of urine (as in small stones), immediate surgery is necessary to prevent further damage to the kidney (HYDRONEPHROSIS). Some kidney stones grow large without symptoms (STAGHORN CALCULUS) and are only discovered when kidney function deteriorates (determined by examining the CREATININE).

LABORATORY EXAMINATIONS:

URINALYSIS – primary laboratory procedure for screening and checking the presence of kidney stones and also the sole determinant to differentiate from URINARYTRACT INFECTION.

CREATININE CLEARANCE DETERMINATION - Blood examination to determine function of the kidney.

ULTRASOUND OF THE KIDNEY – URETER – URINARY BLADDER – the fastest, cheapest and safest way to diagnose kidney stones.

INTRAVENOUS PYELORAM – x-ray procedure involving injections of a contrast media thru the vein and x-rays taken of the kidneys. A lot of people are allergic to this contrast media because of its iodine derivative.

CT SCAN – expensive procedure but do not surpass ultrasound result.

DEFINITIVE PROCEDURE:

NEPHROLITHOTOMY – An opening is made on the flank whichever side is involved extending from the back down to the flank. The kidney is opened via the CALYSIS and the stone is extracted. Some stones cannot be removed due to its size (STAGHORN) and are therefore crushed prior to removal.

EXTRACORPOREAL SHOCK WAVE LITHOTRIPSY – breaking of stone by shockwave. No wound is made. Most are successful but some are unresponsive. Complications range from lacerations of the kidney to blockade. In some centers, success rate is 95%.

BLOODY URINE + INGUINAL PAIN AND SCROTUM (male)

Pain in the flanks associated with bloody urine, inguinal region and radiates to the scrotum in males. Some patients feel numbness of the scrotum, medial side of their thigh and flank.

DIAGNOSIS: URETERAL STONE

ORGAN INVOLVED: ureter (tube that carries urine from the kidney to the urinary bladder)

CAUSE: Stone formation

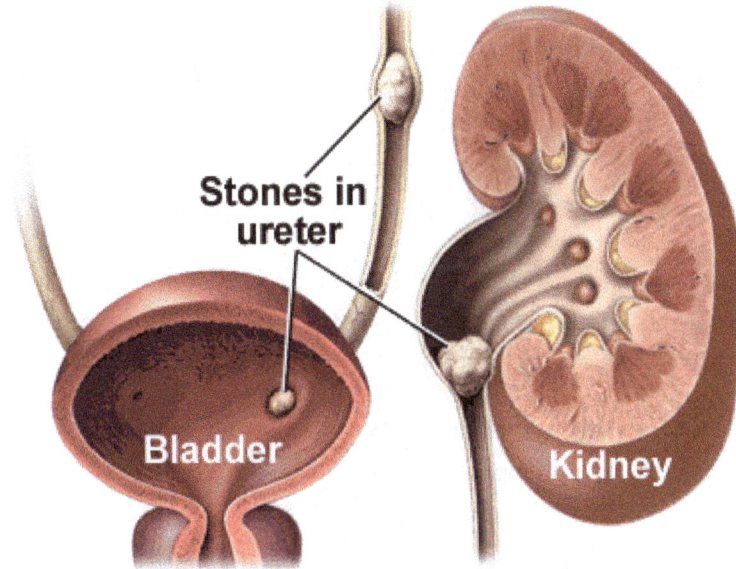

INITIAL TREATMENT:
> BUSCOPAN (Hyoscine butylbromide) 1 tab every 4 hours for pain
> BUCO JUICE
> SAMBUNG tablet 2x a day
> ACALKA (Potassium citrate) tablet 3x a day

ADVICE:

When kidney stone has passed down the ureter, it is more likely to go down to the urinary bladder unless it is lodged in one segment of the tube due to its size. Arrest of the descend causes severe pain but may be relieved by antispasmodic. Due to its damaging effect to the kidney, the blockade of urine (HYDRONEPHROSIS), an immediate surgery is indicated.

LABORATORY EXAMINATIONS:

URINALYSIS - primary diagnostic work up to determine if a stone is present in the urinary tract

CREATININE CLEARANCE – blood examination to determine status of the kidney before surgery

ULTRASOUND OF THE URETER – it is very difficult to maneuver. But in good hands, the stone can be located.

INTRAVENOUS PYELOGRAM - the most accurate x-ray examination to pinpoint the location of the stone in the ureter.

DEFENITIVE TREATMENT:

URETEROLITHOTOMY – surgery is done by an opening on the abdomen whichever side the stone is located with an incision just like that for APPENDECTOMY if it is on the right side at the lower quadrant. The intestinal cavity (PERITONEUM) is not entered but rather retracted to the side and the ureter is found at the back. An opening of the ureter is made and the stone is extracted.

URETERAL LITHOTRIPSY – shock waves pointed at the location of the stone which grinds the stone into fine sand and passed out through urination.

BLOODY URINE + FREQUENCY OF URINATION

Bloody urine associated with frequency of urination, pain during urination, feeling of non-satisfactory urination, abrupt stoppage of urinary stream during urination and the need to find a position in order to urinate (sitting down to urinate)

DIAGNOSIS: URINARY BLADDER STONE

ORGAN INVOLVED: *urinary bladder*

CAUSE: Stone formation

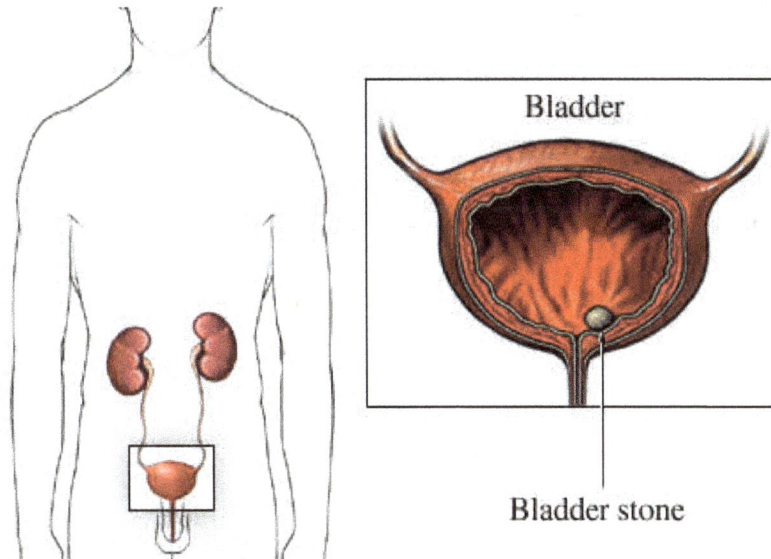

INITIAL TREATMENT:

      ACALKA (Potassium citrate) 1 tab 3x a day
      BUCO JUICE
      SAMBONG 1 tab 3x a day

ADVICE:

Urinary bladder stones may enlarge without symptoms. Some patients have been known to produce stones as large as a golf ball but without symptoms except for urgency (the need to urinate as soon as possible).

LABORATORY EXAMINATIONS:

URINALYSIS - primary diagnostic examination

ULTRASOUND OF THE URINARY BLADDER – readily diagnosed, fast and cheap. Ultrasound of the prostate in male is also done since some patients develop stones due to the enlargement of the prostate.

DEFINITIVE TREATMENT:

OPENCYSTOLITHOTOMY – surgical incision is done at the lower portion of the abdomen. Urinary catheter is inserted to drain out possible bleeding at the incision site.

PANENDOSCOPIC LITHOTRIPSY – an instrument is inserted through the penis and a crushing probe is used to break the stone to small sizes.

EXTRACORPOREAL SOUND WAVE LITHOTRIPSY - a blast of sound is directed towards the urinary bladder to break the stone. This is often done in several courses most especially in big stones.

BLOODY URINE + NO URINARYSTREAM FORCE

Bloody urine associated with difficulty starting urination, frequency of urination, dribbling (droppings of urine), unsatisfactory feeling post urination, long duration of urination and pain even not urinating.

DIAGNOSIS: PROSTATE CANCER

ORGAN INVOLVED: *prostate*

CAUSE: unknown

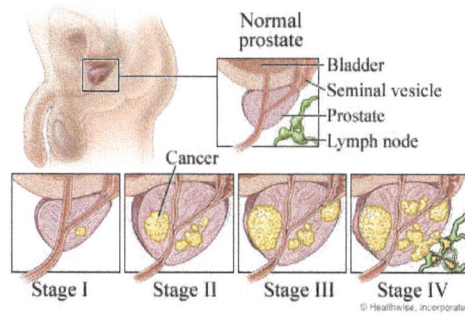

INITIAL TREATMENT: none

ADVICE:

Prostate cancer will start as enlargement of the prostate but will progress into bleeding. Thus, symptoms may present as difficulty starting urination or dribbling in urination, no force in urination and small caliber of stream in urination. Outside of biopsy, diagnosis can be attained by blood examination of PROSTATIC SERUM ASSAY.

LABORATORY EXAMINATION:

URINALYSIS – determines the presence of blood in the urine in minute amount

ULTRASOUND OF THE PROSTATE – will indicate enlargement of the prostate

PROSTATIC SERUM ASSAY - determines the presence of prostate cancer

ENDOCOSPIC PROSTATIC BIOPSY – through a tube with light source, the prostate is visualized via the penile shaft and a piece of tissue is removed and examined in the laboratory.

DEFINITIVE TREATMENT:

PROSTATECTOMY – the removal of the whole prostate through open surgery or endoscopy. Erection will be sacrificed and sexual life will be dampened.

CHEMOTHERAPY – dismal results

RADIOTHERAPY – dismal results

BLOOD IN THE SPUTUM

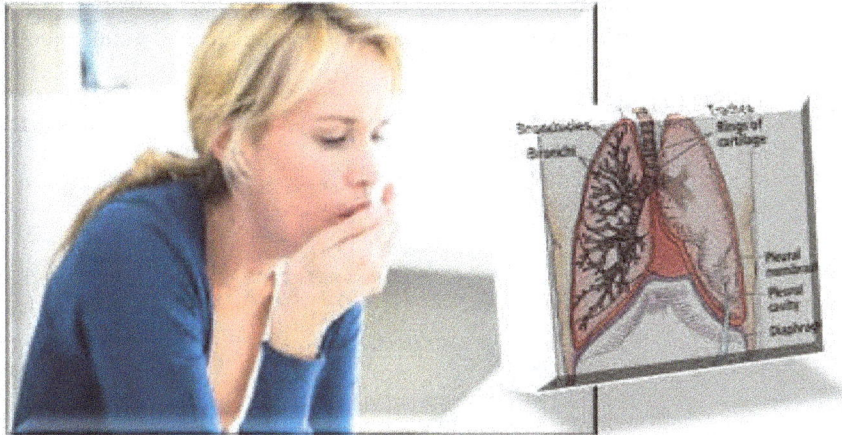

Blood in the sputum is usually attributed to TUBERCULOSIS OF THE LUNGS. But there are a lot of diseases that manifest as blood in the sputum and should be differentiated from it. The objective of this chapter is to differentiate the symptoms related to bloody sputum in order to pinpoint the real cause. The reader is cautioned that definitive diagnosis rests on the acuity of the physician, and thus, the need for consultation and diagnostic work up could not be overemphasized.

Bleeding from the gums, tooth, tongue and tonsils can be readily detected by an untrained eye. Gurgling of cold water is the only treatment for them. However, blood that is vomited should be differentiated from blood in the sputum; in that, the former usually comes after severe vomiting and not coughing. This also needs immediate admission to the hospital as nothing could help the patient at home.

BLOODY SPUTUM + COUGH + AFTERNOON FEVER

Cough that produces yellowish phlegm with blood streaks will result to a massive bleeding (HEMOPTYSIS) is associated with afternoon fever, loss of weight, no appetite and general body malaise.

DIAGNOSIS: PULMONARY TUBERCULOSIS

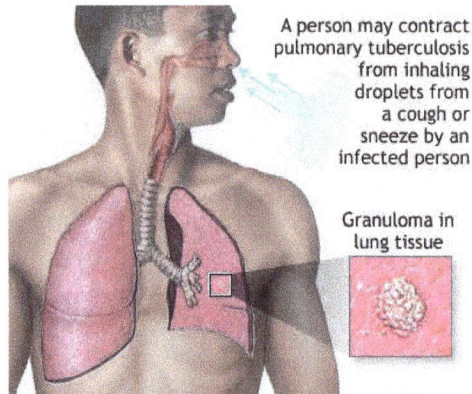

A person may contract pulmonary tuberculosis from inhaling droplets from a cough or sneeze by an infected person

Granuloma in lung tissue

ORGAN INVOLVED: *lungs*

CAUSE: Mycobacterium tuberculosis

INITIAL TREATMENT:
CYCLOKAPRON (Tranexamic acid) 1 tab 3x a day for 1 week
AMBROXOL (Mucosolvan) 75 mg 1 tab once a day

ADVICE:

Tuberculosis of the lungs is contagious through direct inhalation. Therefore, the infection cannot be taken from utensils such as spoons and plates unless directly used from the mouth of infected individual to the receiver. Treatment should be continuous until Chest x-ray shows complete healing. Tuberculosis is also found in the skin, intestines, liver and all other parts of the body and most often mislead physician to think of cancer by its presence. Biopsy of the tumor is the only way to differentiate cancer from Tuberculosis. Follow up chest x-rays should be done every three months in order to substantiate complete healing.

LABORATORY EXAMINITAIONS:

CHEST X-RAY – determines the presence of cavitations and lesions in the upper portion of the lungs

SPUTUM EXAM FOR ACID FAST BACILLI – three consecutive examination of the sputum taken early in the morning placed in a wide mouthed bottle.

CYTOLOGIC EXAMINATION OF SPUTUM – use to rule out the possibility of cancer.

DEFINITIVE TREATMENT:

MYRIN P FORTE 1 tab 3x a day for 3 months

BLOODY SPUTUM + LOST OF WEIGHT+ CHEST PAINS

Bloody sputum usually proceeded by loss of weight, history of smoking, and body malaise then followed by gnawing pain on the chest or at the back. Some patients do not manifest any blood in their sputum at all. Others are accidentally discovered on routine chest x-ray.

DIAGNOSIS: LUNG CANCER

ORGAN INVOLVED: *lungs*

CAUSE: strongly related to smoking

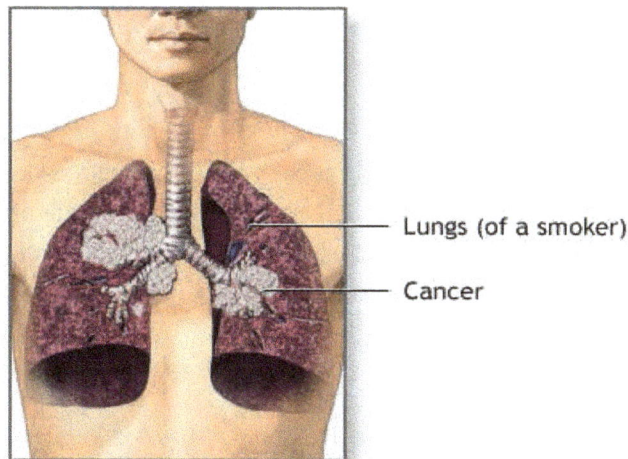

Lungs (of a smoker)

Cancer

INITIAL TREATMENT: none

ADVICE:

Lung cancer has no prevention except refraining from smoking starting at young age. When discovered by X –ray, patient has only a few months to live with or without surgery, chemotherapy or radiation. Prolongation of life through these modalities does not improve quality of life. Patient would be miserable throughout these remaining days much more aggravated by these modalities.

LABORATORY EXAMINATIONS:

CHEST X-RAY – is the most common diagnostic exam that discovers the lesion. They would appear as single or multiple small rounded lesions on the lungs that are referred to as "coin lesion" by radiologists.

BRONCHIAL WASHINGS – through bronchoscopy (a fiber-optic tube used to visualize the inside of the bronchus), pieces of the bronchus are taken for laboratory examination. The tube is inserted direct to the bronchus with patient half-awake or generally anesthetized. Diagnostic accuracy is minimal if the lesion is in the lungs and not in the tubes (bronchus).

CYTOLOGY EXAM OF SPUTUM – some lung cancers can be diagnosed through this method. This is done by collecting all the sputum expectorated by the patient in 24 hours. Lung cancer detection is not accurate. Many are missed by this method.

CT SCAN – a diagnostic work up to determine the respectability of the lesion (whether patient can benefit by radical surgery). Biopsy of the lesion may be done with the guide of this modality.

DEFINITIVE TREATMENT:

TOTAL LOBECTOMY – removal of the entire lung or a lobe of the lung on one side through an opening of the chest called *THORACOTOMY*. Lung capacity of the remaining lung is often measured prior to surgery to determine whether it can support patient post-surgery. Patients with lung impairment like Bronchial asthma, Emphysema, Chronic obstructive lung disease aside from lung cancer would not benefit from this surgery. He would become a LUNG CRIPPLE and would need VENTILATING MACHINE to support him the rest of his days. This surgery may prolong his life 4 - 6 months more.

CHEMOTHERAPY – dismal results
RADIOTHERAPY – dismal results.

BLOODY SPUTUM + SEVERE FORCEFUL COUGH

Bloody sputum associated with severe cough appearing right after a forceful coughing. This may lead to expectoration of massive amount of blood. History of smoking can be extracted from the patient.

DIAGNOSIS: ACUTE BRONCHIECTASIS

ORGAN INVLOVED: *bronchus*

CAUSE: laceration of the bronchus due to forceful coughing.

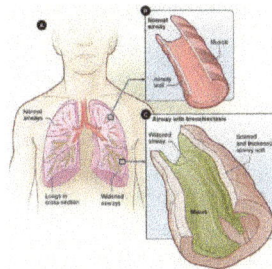

INTIAL TREATMENT: *Rush to the hospital*
ALLOW PATIENT TO COUGH BLOOD OUT – clotted blood inside the bronchus is much more dangerous than those cough out. This could block the airway.
Cold drinks and cold compress on the chest may help.
HEMOSTAN (Tranexamic acid) 500 mg 1 cap 3x a day

ADVICE:
Irritation of the throat is usually the cause of forceful coughing. Unabated coughing results in the tearing of the mucosal lining of the bronchus. If bleeding does not stop with blood clotting injections, bronchoscopy is necessary to fulgurate the bleeding points.

LABORATORY EXAMINATION:
CHEST X-RAY - to determine other source of bleeding in the lungs

BRONCHOSCOPY – it is used as a diagnostic as well as therapeutic. Visualization of the bleeding point is the best way to control it. The procedure is very difficult.

CT SCAN – can be done if the patient is not pulmonary distress. It does not help in the emergency procedure.

DEFINITIVE TREATMENT:

BRONCHOSCOPY – visualization of bleeding points need an experienced Pulmonologist. In good hands, procedure is easy and fast. Cauterization of the bleeding points is the only procedure that can be done to stop bleeding.

THORACOTOMY – opening of the chest cavity and looking for the bleeding points as seen in chest x-ray. This is a very radical procedure. Anesthesia of the patient is very difficult.

VOMITING BLOOD (HEMATEMESIS)

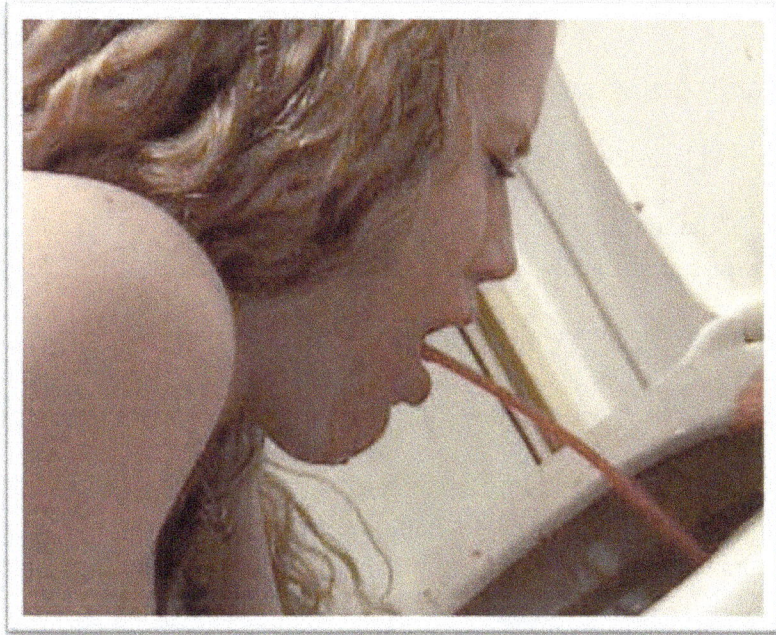

Blood in the vomitus usually comes from the teeth, gums, tonsils and pharynx. They are often caused by trauma and could be explained readily. Treatment often consists only of ice or cold water to suppress bleeding. What is more alarming is when a person suddenly vomits blood of profuse quantity. This often causes panic to the person and to the relatives. The next chapter deals on the causes of this disease. It should be borne in mind that these diseases require utmost discernment whether the blood comes from the lungs or from the GASTROINTESTINAL TRACT.

The arrow indicates the chronological sequence of happening (i.e. vomiting followed by blood in the vomit)

VOMITING ➡️ BLOOD VOMIT

Severe vomiting or wrenching with yellowish saliva or food followed by appearance of blood in the vomit.

DIAGNOSIS: PHARYNGO-ESOPHAGEAL LACERATION

CAUSE: a forceful vomiting lacerates the mucosa of the pharynx or esophagus

INITIAL TREATMENT: Ask patient to drink ice-cold water until vomit does not contain blood. Water could be substituted with soft-drinks or any juice.

ADVICE: Forceful vomiting causes avulsion of the pharyngo-esophageal mucosa (lining) which contain abundant blood vessels. If the avulsion is small laceration, the bleeding may not be so profuse. It would stop in 5 to 10 minutes. If the vomitus persistently contains blood, consultation should be done.

There are diseases that predispose a person to vomit blood. UREMIA (kidney failure), LIVER CIRRHOSIS (LIVER FAILURE), ANEMIA, LUEKEMIA and cancer of the esophagus are some of these diseases. If vomiting of blood occurs for the first time, lab exams should be done to rule out these diseases.

LABORATORY EXAMINATIONS:

CREATININE – for UREMIA

SGPT – for liver failure

CBC – for anemia

PERIPHERAL SMEAR – for leukemia

PLATELET COUNT – for blood related diseases

ESOPHAGOGRAM – for cancer of the esophagus

DEFINITIVE TREATMENT:

ESOPHAGOSCOPY (GASTROSCOPY) – a fiber-optic tube is inserted into the mouth to examine the whole length of the esophagus. Fulguration (burning) of bleeding points can be done with this instrument. Before the advent of this instrument, exploration of the esophagus was usually done by surgery with a wound made on the chest extending from the back to the front. This was indicated in patients who develop massive bleeding from the esophagus.

DRUNKEN SEVERE VOMITING BLOOD

After a bout of drinking, a person vomits profusely followed by profuse bleeding from the mouth.

DIAGNOSIS: MALLORY-WEISS SYNDROME

CAUSE: linear laceration of the mucosa at the junction of the esophagus and stomach.

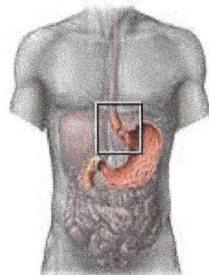

A Mallory-Weiss tear is a tear in the mucosal layer at the junction of the esophagus and stomach

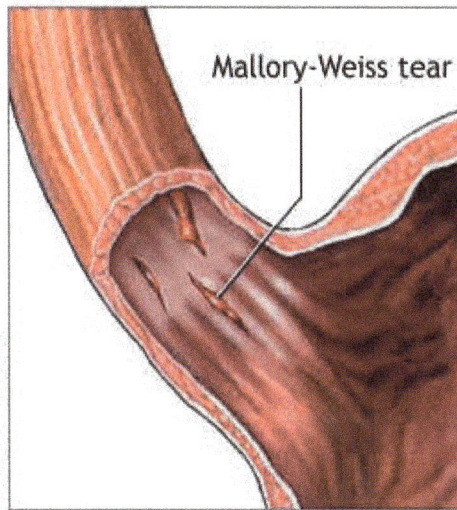

Mallory-Weiss tear

INITIAL TREATMENT:

Ask the patient to drink ice-cold water until he can be brought to the hospital. Very sweet juice or drinks will help in stopping nausea and vomiting.

ADVICE:

Drinking alcohol stimulates the GASTROINTESTINAL TRACT and cause hiccups. This is often followed with severe vomiting. Forceful vomiting causes abrupt opening of the GASTRO-ESOPHAGEAL JUNCTION (point between the lower-most portion of the esophagus and the upper portion of the stomach) that in turn causes laceration/tearing of the mucosa (lining of the esophagus). Blood vessels found underneath the mucosa are torn causing massive bleeding and vomiting of blood.

LABORATORY EXAMINATION:

ESOPHAGOSCOPY – it is both diagnostic as well a therapeutic. In some cases, due to massive bleeding, the procedure may not stop the bleeding due to visual difficulty.

DEFINITIVE TREATMENT:

EXPLORATION OF THE ESOPHAGUS – This is done by making an opening on the abdomen by surgery, going thru the stomach and suturing the bleeding points in the gastro-esophageal junction.

NOSE BLEEDING

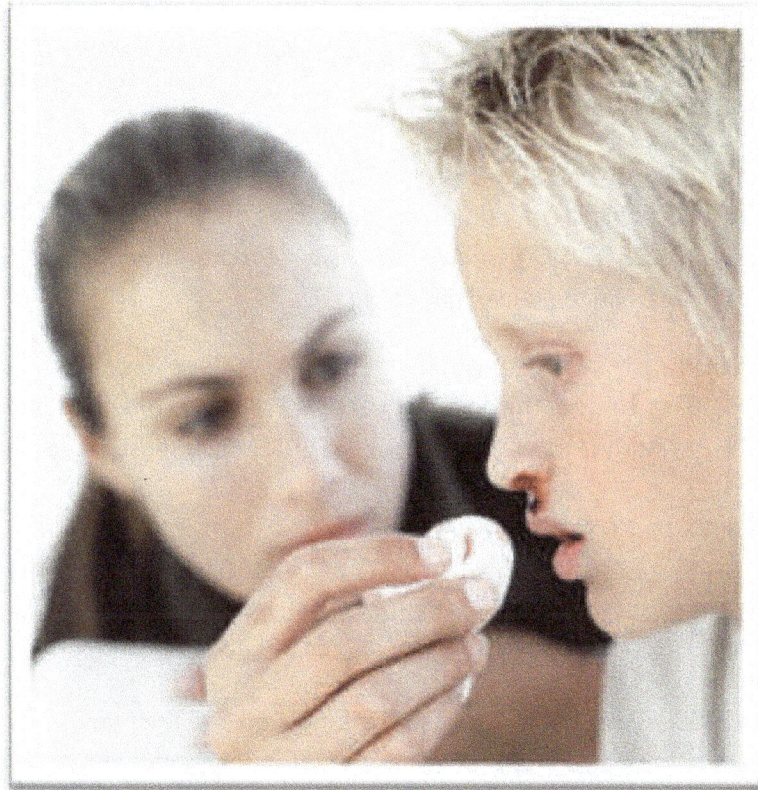

Nose bleeding may be spontaneous or can be caused by trauma. Over all, allowing the blood to come out through the nose is the best way to prevent difficulty of breathing. Preventing blood to pass through the nose and allowing it to pass through the back of the mouth may cause blockade of the airway.

SPONTANEOUS NOSE BLEEDING - In children, the most common cause is laceration of the superficially located blood vessels in the turbinates of the nose injured when they pick their nose. Some children have the history of liniment application direct to the nose or the use of mentholated inhalers.

TRAUMATIZED NOSE BLEEDING – mauling straight to the nose causes fracture of the nasal cartilage and the accompanying laceration of the turbinates inside the nose

INITIAL TREATMENT:
COLD COMPRESS ON THE FOREHEAD AND NASAL BRIDGE
GURGLE OF ICE COLD WATER
HEMOSTAN 500 mg 1 cap 3x a day for 5 days

ADVICE: Spontaneous nose bleeding is sometimes the symptoms of systemic illness like LEUKEMIA, SICKLE CELLANEMIA, UREMIA, and HYPERTENSION. These diseases have to be ruled out with the use of laboratory examinations. Treatment is based on the underlying cause.

LABORATORY EXAMINATIONS:
PERIPHERAL SMEAR – to rule out the possibility of LUEKEMIA, and other blood related diseases
BLOOD PRESSURE DETERMINATION – to rule out HYPERTENSION most especially in the older age group
CREATININE DETERMINATION – to rule out UREMIA
PLATELET COUNT – to rule out the possibility of clotting mechanism diseases like DENGUE
CT SCAN OF THE CRANIUM – done to rule out the possibility of brain injury as in trauma.

DEFINITIVE TREATMENT:
PACKING OF THE NOSE – strips of gauze bandage is inserted into the nose
POSTCHOANAL PACKING – a pack of gauze is inserted thru the mouth and packed just at the back of the nose above the pharynx
VITAMIN K INJECTION - to help in the clotting mechanism

TREATMENT OF THE UNDERLYING DISEASES

BLOOD IN ANUS AND STOOLS

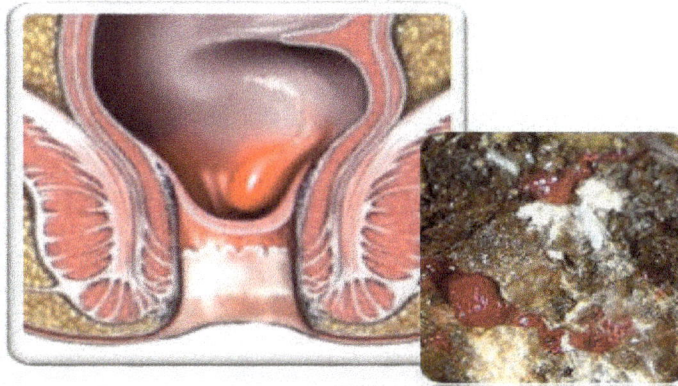

Bloody stools or fresh blood from the anus signify lower intestinal bleeding as compared to bleeding in the upper portion of the intestine wherein, the blood becomes black due to reaction of the stomach acidity to it. Thus, fresh blood in the stools directs the reader's attention to the diseases found near the anus, such as, in the large intestines and the anus itself. Diagnosis in the clinical setting is usually accomplished by doing rectal examination and visual examination of the anus. No other diagnostic exam could surpass this outside of doing colonoscopy that entails lot of expense and time. If by no other means, the patient could not examine himself for such lesions in the anus, examination by a doctor should be the primary objective to attain diagnosis. Simply put, no exact diagnosis no effective treatment.

The objective of this chapter is for the reader to know the different diseases affecting the anus, when to self-medicate, as well as, when to go for checkup. It also discusses the medications that could be used temporarily to alleviate symptoms and to understand his physician why he recommends such, and such diagnostic work up, the recommended treatment and the following complications that may result with or without treatment.

FRESH BLOOD from the Anus

Fresh blood coming out of the anus associated with pain in the anal opening and usually following bowel movement of big, form, hard stools and no history of hemorrhoids

DIAGNOSIS: ANAL FISSURES

ORGAN INVOLVED: *anal canal*

CAUSE: laceration of the anal mucosa

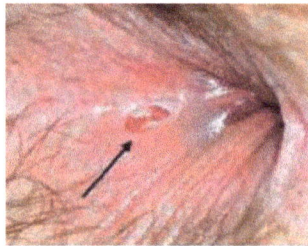

Anal Fissure

INITIAL TREATMENT:

HOT SITZ – sitting on a warm water in basin mixed with salt
HEMOSTAN (Tranexamic acid) 500 mg 1 cap 3x a day for 7 days
FAKTU 1 SUPP daily at night for 7 days

ADVICE:

Most anal bleeding due to fissures stops on its own even without treatment. But the complications are more of a problem than the disease itself. This usually leads to FISTULA IN ANU if untreated or injury is repeated several times. Prevention like taking laxatives *(SENOKOT TABLET DAILY)* and /or eating papaya every day is very important. If symptoms persist, consultation with a doctor is a must to determine the presence of malignant lesions.

LABORATORY EXAMINATION: none

DEFINITIVE TREATMENT:

PROCTOSIGMOIDOSCOPY – A diagnostic as well as curative to determine the cause and fulgurate the bleeding points.

FRESH BLOOD IN THE ANUS + ABDOMINAL PAIN

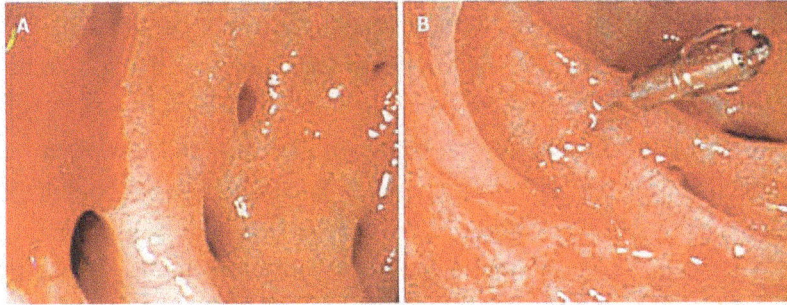

Fresh blood in the anus with no history of hemorrhoids or pain during bowel movement. There is a crampy abdominal pain in the left lower quadrant prior to the bowel movement or the urge to move one's bowel.

DIAGNOSIS: BLEEDING COLONIC DIVERTICULUM

ORGAN INVOLVED: colon

CAUSE: weakening of the wall of the colon and formation of a sac-like deformity

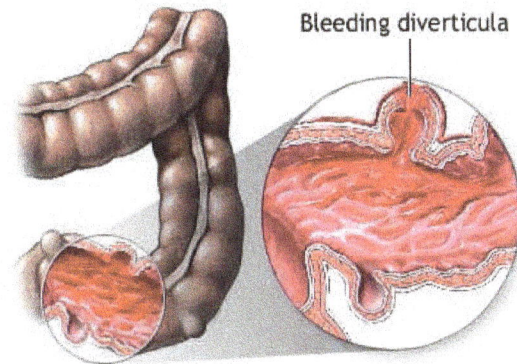

Bleeding diverticula

INITIAL TREATMENT: *NONE*

ADVICE:

More often than not, this diagnosis is a differential diagnosis to other illnesses.

It is an incidental finding in a BARIUM ENEMA rather than a disease being searched for. But, it is one of the causes of fresh blood passing through the anus.

ADIVERTICULUM is an out-pouching or the formation of a sack on the wall of neither the intestine the cause of which is unknown nor the force that causes it. Because of the abundance of blood vessels in this sack, bleeding is more common in any state of the stools: loose bowel movement, constipation, and normal stool. It is also the site of infection mimicking ACUTE APPENDICITIS if it is located on the right side portion of the large intestine, TWISTED OVARIAN CYST if it is located on the left, PELVIC INFLAMMATORY DISEASE if it is located in the SIGMOID portion of the large intestine just below the urinary bladder.

LABORATORY EXAMINATION:

BARIUM ENEMIA – applied to determine other diseases such as malignancy in the large intestine. Milk-like substance is pumped direct to the anus and x-rays are taken while the patient holds the substance.

COLONOSCOPY – can miss the presence of a diverticulum most especially when the opening of the sack is minute and cannot be detected visually.

DEFINITIVE TREATMENT:

None, unless life threatening like in severe infection of the diverticulum (DIVERTICULITIS) and severe bleeding in which case:

COLONIC RESECTION – removal of a segment of the large intestine with preservation of the continuity of the intestine (end to end anastomosis)

DROPS OF BLOOD IN TOILET BOWL

Bleeding from preexisting hemorrhoids triggered by hard form stools usually noted as fresh blood in tissue paper post defecation or drops of blood in the toilet bowl.

DIAGNOSIS: BLEEDING HEMORRHOIDS

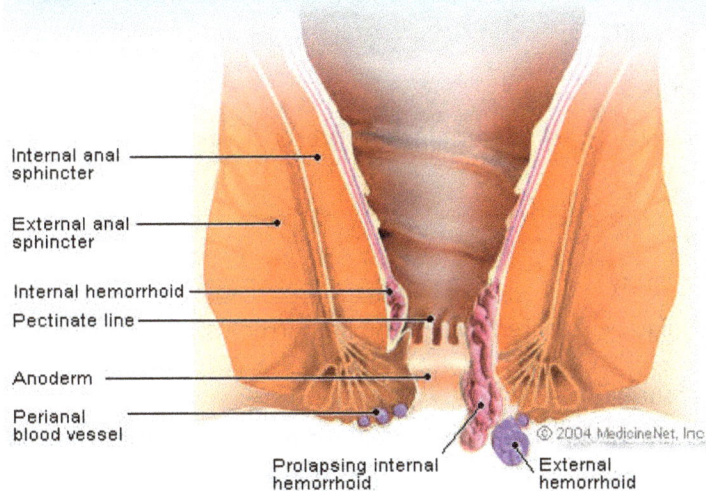

Formation of hemorrhoids

ORAGAN INVOLVED: *anus*

CAUSE: Bleeding of thrombosed hemorrhoids.

INITIAL TREATMENT:

HOT SITZ bath – sitting on a basin of warm water for 15 minutes 2x a day

FAKTU SUPP stick daily for 7 days
DAFLON 500 mg 1 cap 3x a day for 7 days

ADVICE:

Hemorrhoids are commonly caused by pregnancy, carrying heavy weight, obesity, chronic constipation and, never due to spicy foods. Non- bleeding hemorrhoids may not need treatment. But they are the most common cause of FISTULA IN ANU.

Life may not be affected even without treatment of hemorrhoids. But some hemorrhoids may be the only symptom of an underlying malignancy in the large intestine. Thus, specimen post hemorrhoidectomy is always sent to the laboratory for HISTOPATH (microscopic examination of a tissue) to determine any signs of malignancy.

LABORATORY EXAMINATION

PROCTOSIGMOIDOSCOPY – to determine any presence of malignancy in the upper portion of the large intestine

DEFINITIVE TREATMENT:

HEMORRHOIDECTOMY:

White head technique – total removal of the hemorrhoids.

Complications of surgery are the following:
1. Anal stricture – anal canal is greatly diminished causing difficulty in bowel movement.
2. Wet anus – severe exposure of the lining of the anus causing wetness of the underwear and subsequent smell.

Diamond technique – it is a partial removal of the hemorrhoids in different quadrants of the anal introitus.

Complications:
1. recurrence – formation of hemorrhoids in other part of the anus
2. FISTULA IN ANU – formation of canals in areas of surgery.

Chapter Three

FEVER

FEVER

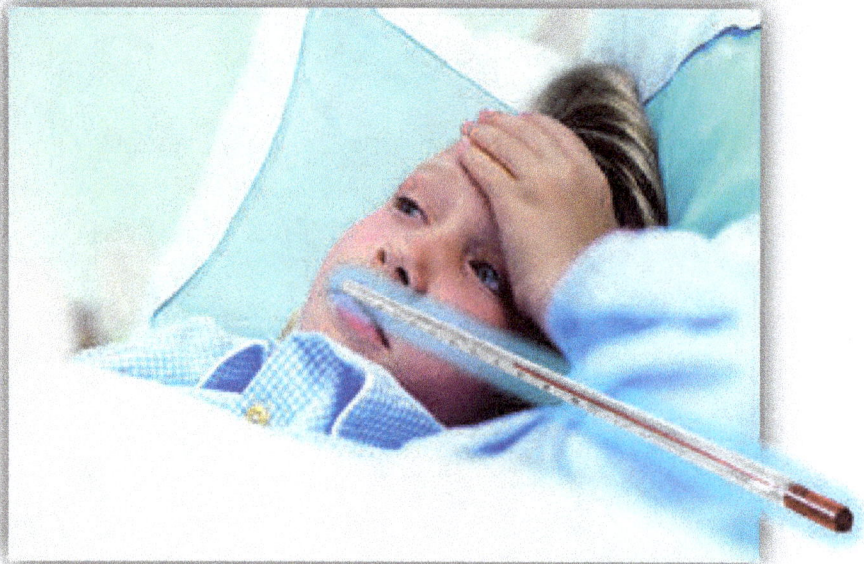

Normally, even by itself alone, the origin or cause of fever could be determined. Some of the characteristics of the fever, namely: when it starts, how long it stays, when it recurs, and what time of the day it occurs, give away the diagnosis. Knowing the characteristics of the fever give some hints to the reader when to seek consultation and when to self-medicate. Understanding the doctor's recommendation enables the patient to be enthusiastic with the prescribed medications despite the cost.

The reader is cautioned not to rely too much on his own observation. Remittent fever may be elusive to monitor. Spiking fever may not be spiking at all, when observed at a regular interval. So, monitoring should be done in about 2 days before qualifying a fever, as such.

The taking of medications such as PARACETAMOL disrupts the normal curve of fever. If these medications are taken, exact monitoring and determination of the character of the fever may be lost. The time of intake of medication should also be taken into consideration.

AFTERNOON FEVER

Fever usually occurring in the afternoon or late in the afternoon associated with body malaise, loss of weight, chronic cough and chest and back pains.

DIAGNOSIS: TUBERCULOSIS OF THE LUNGS

ORGAN INVOLVED: *lungs*

CAUSE: Mycobacterium tuberculosis

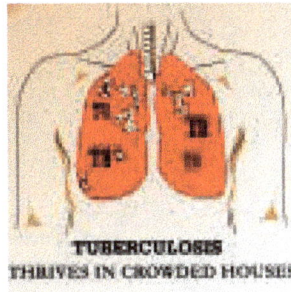

TUBERCULOSIS
THRIVES IN CROWDED HOUSES

INITIAL TREATMENT:

PARACETAMOL 500 mg 1 tab every 4 hours for fever

ADVICE:

Tuberculosis of the lungs may not manifest as blood in sputum or even marked lost weight. Most individuals discovered with Tuberculosis have no symptoms even cough. Routine chest x-ray is the only method of detecting symptom-less Tuberculosis.

LABORATORY EXAMINATION:

CHEST X-RAY: should be done yearly most especially for people who live with individuals with known Tuberculosis of the lungs. Repeat x-ray should be done after treatment to determine eradication of the bacteria.

SPUTUM EXAM FOR ACID FAST BACILLI – collection of sputum in a 24 hr. period and submission of the specimen in the laboratory. This will identify the bacterium responsible for Tuberculosis

DEFINITIVE TREATMENT:

MYRIN –P FORTE tablet 3x a day for 3 months

FEVER WITH CHILLS

Remittent fever (non-stop fever) accompanied by chills, headache, frequency of urination, flank pain or pain during urination

DIAGNOSIS: URINARY TRACT INFECTION

ORGAN INVOLVED: *kidney, urinary bladder*

CAUSE: Infection of the above organs

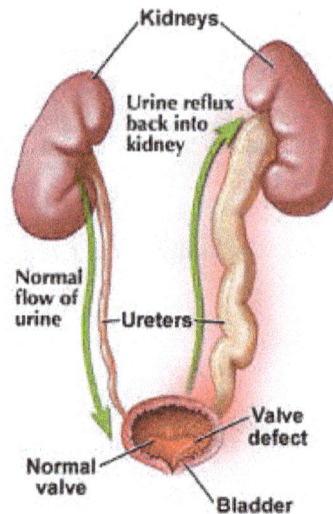

INITIAL TREATMENT:

PARACETAMOL 500 mg tablet every 4 hours for fever

ADVICE:

This is common in women most especially child bearing age and young adults. Diagnosis is often directed to the kidney when flank pains or abdominal pains accompany the symptoms. The absence of this symptom often will lead one to another diagnosis.

LABORATORY EXAMINATION:

URINALYSIS – presence of pus cells of more than 6+ with red blood cells (RBC)

DEFINITIVE TREATMENT:

TEQUIN (Gatifloxacin) 400 mg tablet single dose for the next 3 days if symptoms persist.

FEVER + WATERY STOOLS + HEADACHE

Fever preceded by loose bowel movement in about 3 - 5 days associated with headaches, body malaise and bitter taste. Pulse is unusually slow during the febrile period.

DIAGNOSIS: ACUTE TYPHOID FEVER

ORGAN INVOLVED: *small intestine*

CAUSE: Salmonella typhosi

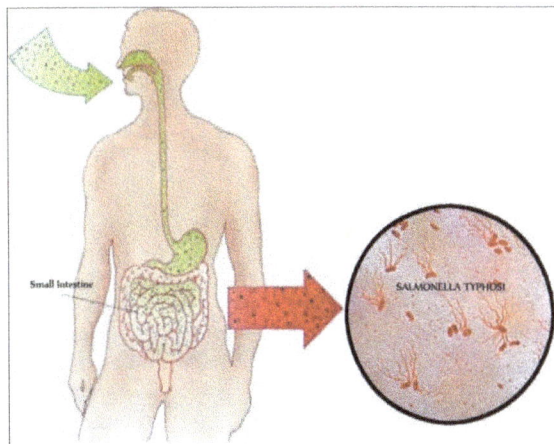

INITIAL TREATMENT:

MEFENAMIC ACID 500 mg tablet every 4 hours for headache

PARACETAMOL 500 mg tablet every 4 hours for fever

ADVICE:

Typhoid fever may start with loose bowel movement without fever. 3-5 days after the LBM ceases, headaches, fever and body malaise may start. Fever is usually noted to be high grade and continuous.

LABORATORY EXAMINATION:

WIDAL TEST – blood examination which detects presence of Typhoid in the blood

TYPHIDOT – blood exam which is more accurate and fast than WIDAL TEST but more expensive

DEFINITIVE TREATMENT:

CHLORAMPHENICOL 500 mg 1 cap 4x a day for 10 days **OR**

OFLOXACIN 200 mg tablet 2x a day for 7 days

FEVER + RASHES ON LEGS

Dengue fever is characterized by: Fever
Rash
Muscle and
joint pains

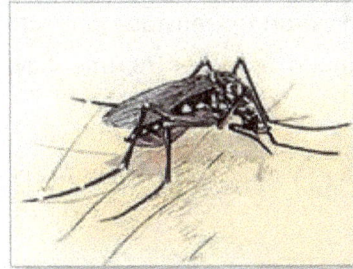

Aedes aegypti mosquito

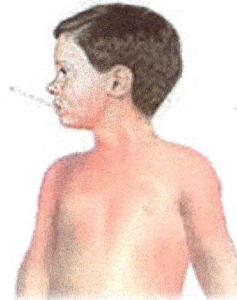

High-   grade fever
usually above 40 followed by the appearance of rashes on the legs and arms. Face, hands and feet are noted
to be reddish than the rest of the body and are cold despite the presence of fever.

DIAGNOSIS: DENGUE FEVER

ORGAN INVOLVED: *blood*

CAUSE: viral infection from mosquito bite

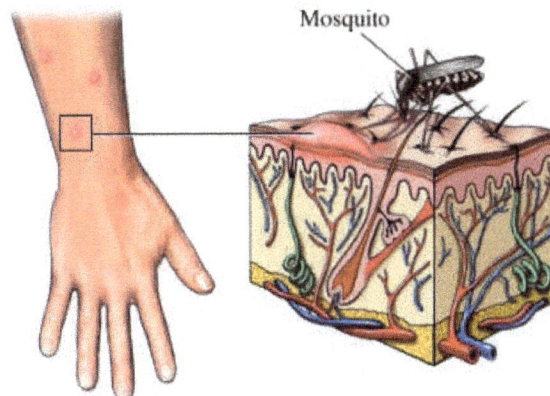

Mosquito

INITIAL TREATMENT:

PARACETAMOL 500 mg tablet every 4 hours or syrup 1 tsp. every 4 hours

ADVICE:

Treatment of DENGUE consists of monitoring the platelet of the patient at the hospital setting. When the platelet count drops to 30,000 it is an indication to transfuse platelet concentrate or fresh whole blood if the former is not available. There is no vaccination or other treatment available.

LABORATORY EXAMINATION:

PLATELET COUNT – normal is above 120,000. Any rapid decrease in the count indicates DENGUE FEVER.

DENGUE RAPID TEST – recently launched exam for dengue but is not 100% accurate. Some may give false negative results or false positive results.

HEMOGLOBIN AND HEMATOCRIT – blood concentration test necessary to monitor decrease of platelet. They are also necessary in the transfusion procedure.

DEFINITIVE TREATMENT:

PLATELET CONCENTRATE – transfused to the patient in the event where platelet count drops down below 30,000.

FEVER + COLD + COUGH

Fever followed by colds and cough with body malaise. In children, fever is accompanied by anorexia, vomiting and cold clammy perspiration.

DIAGNOSIS: ACUTE INFLUENZA

ORGAN INLVOLVED: upper respiratory tract (nose, pharynx, bronchus)
CAUSE: viral infection of the upper respiration tract

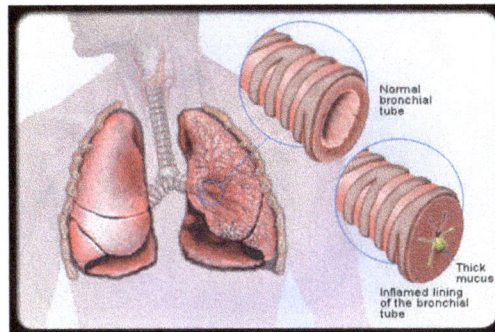

INITIAL TREATMENT:

For children:

> PARACETAMOL SYRUP 1 tsp. every 4 hrs.
> DIMETAPP SYRUP 1 tsp. 3x a day for 5 days
> TOCLASE SYRUP 1 tsp. 3x a day for 5 days

For adult:

> PARACETAMOL 500 mg tablet every 4 hours for fever
> MYONAL (Eperisone) tablet 3x a day for 5 days for muscle pains
> AMBROXOL 75 mg tablet daily for cough
> NASATHERA tablet 3x a day for 5 days for colds

ADVICE:

Acute influenza ends by itself without treatment. Medications are given to abate symptoms. There is still no drug to eradicate viral infection in the upper respiratory. Thus, prevention of the dreaded complications of acute influenza (pneumonia) is of utmost importance. Warm bath or shower, avoidance from exposure to cold and prevention of the rise of temperature are the objective in the management of this illness.

LABORATORY EXAMINATION:

COMPLETE BLOOD COUNT – done to determine whether cause of fever is not bacterial infection.

DEFINITIVE TREATMENT: *none*

FEVER + YELLOWISH DISCOLORATION OF THE EYES

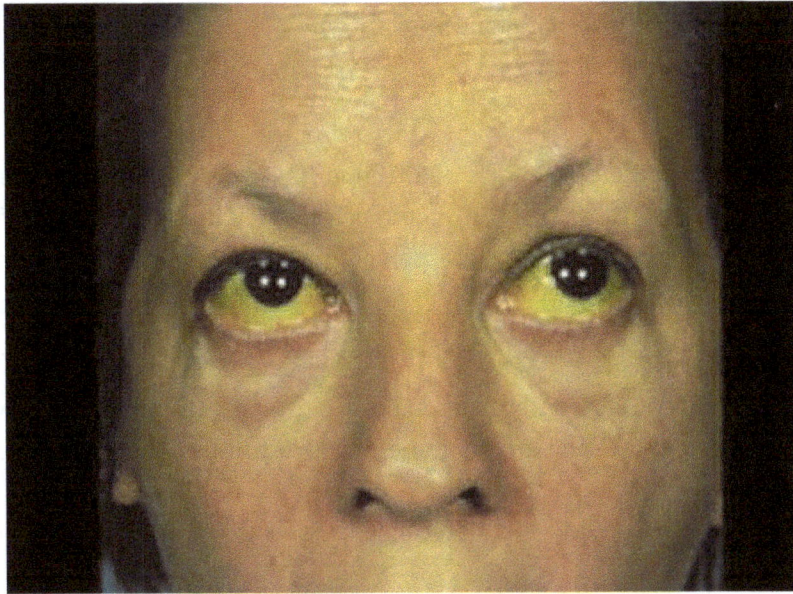

Fever followed by yellowish eyes, body malaise, epigastric fullness and itchiness of the entire body

DIAGNOSIS: HEPATITIS

ORGAN INVOLVED: *liver*

CAUSE: Hepatitis viral infection (A-B-C)

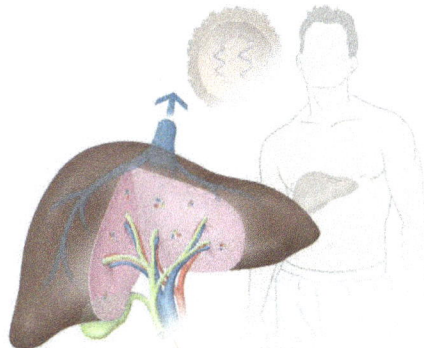

INITIAL TREATMENT :

    PARACETAMOL 500 mg tablet every 4 hours for fever

    ESSENTIAL FORTE tablet 3x a day – vitamins for the liver

    CETIRIZINE tablet daily – for itchiness

ADVICE:

    Hepatitis may come from different sources of infection (saliva droplets for A, blood transfusion for B and C). Of the three kinds of hepatitis, hepatitis B is the most dreaded disease because of the possibility of causing cancer (HEPATOMA). All are self-limiting disease and may resolve itself without treatment. Antiviral medications are still not available for hepatitis A.

LABORATORY EXAMINATIONS:

    HEPATITIS B SURFACE ANTIGEN – determines exposure to Hepatitis B infection or vaccination. Most foreign countries require overseas foreign workers to be negative to this test. A person who is positive to this test will not be employed.

    HEPATITIS B ANTI-ANTIGEN (IGM) – it determines the presence of active infection or recently acquired immunity.

    SGPT / SGOT – blood examinations to determine liver function

    ULTRASOUND OF THE LIVER – GALL BLADDER- COMMON BILE DUCT – PANCREAS: done to determine the possibility of other causes of jaundice (yellowish discoloration)

DEFINITIVE TREATMENT: for HEPATITIS B only

    LAMIVUDINE tablet 2x a day for 10-14 days

FEVER + JAUNDICE + ABDOMINALPAIN + CHILLS

High-grade fever associated with yellowish color of skin and eyes, severe abdominal pains localized in the epigastric area and chills.

DIAGNOSIS: ACUTE CHOLANGITIS

ORGAN INLVOLVED: *common bile duct*

CAUSE: swelling of the tubes that deliver bile from the liver to the intestines due to infection.

INITIAL TREATMENT:
   PARACETAMOL 500 mg tablet every 4 hours
   CEFUROXIME 500 mg tablet 3x a day

ADVICE:
   This is an emergency situation. Because of infection of the tubes (common bile duct), obstruction to the flow of bile destroys the liver at the same time allowing infection to spread all over the body. The only treatment is to relieve the obstruction by surgery. Fighting infection by antibiotics does not help.

LABORATORY EXAMINATIONS:
   ULTRASOUND OF THE LIVER, GALL BLADDER, COMMON BILE DUCT AND PANCREAS – yellowish discoloration of the eyes and skin has so many causes. It is only through this examination that definite diagnosis could be accomplished in a short time.

ALKALINE PHOSPHATASE – blood exam that determines any disease found only in the common bile duct and infection is one of them.

DEFINITIVE TREATMENT:

EXPLORATORY LAPAROTOMY – a general term used to describe surgical opening of the abdomen to determine the cause of an illness.

CHOLECYSTOSTOMY – it is a relief of the bile obstruction by opening the gall bladder and draining it out through a skin opening. Thus, it is a temporary procedure just to relieve the obstruction. A definite surgery will follow when the patient passes the crisis.

CHOLEDOCHOSTOMY – relief of the bile obstruction by re-channeling the bile flow into the outside by:

1. T-TUBE CHOLEDOCHOSTOMY – inserting a tube into the common bile duct and draining it out thru a small skin incision.
2. CHOLEDOCO-DUODENOSTOMY – short circuiting the common bile duct by attaching it direct to the duodenum – a portion of small intestine next to the stomach
3. CHOLEDOCO-JEJUNOSTOMY – short-circuiting the common bile duct by attaching it direct to the jejunum – a part of the small intestine distal to the stomach.

FEVER + COUGH + DIFFICULTY OF BREATHING

Fever of several days associated with cough and body malaise followed by chest pains and difficulty of breathing. Cough usually productive of yellowish phlegm and may initiate pain in the chest

DIAGNOSIS: ACUTE LOBAR PNEUMONIA

ORGAN INVOLVED: *lungs*

CAUSE: bacterial infection of the lungs

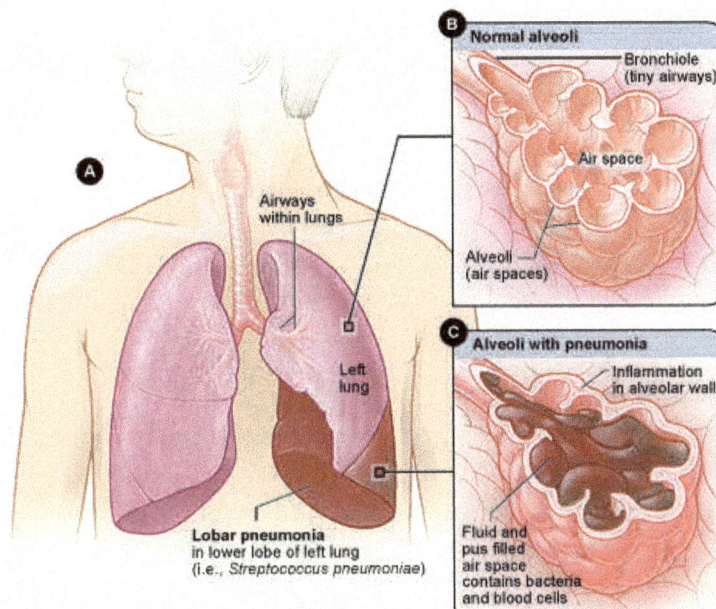

A.
Airways within lungs

Left lung

Lobar pneumonia
in lower lobe of left lung
(i.e., *Streptococcus pneumoniae*)

B. Normal alveoli
Bronchiole (tiny airways)
Air space
Alveoli (air spaces)

C. Alveoli with pneumonia
Inflammation in alveolar wall
Fluid and pus filled air space contains bacteria and blood cells

INITIAL TREATMENT:

PARACETAMOL 500 mg tablet every 4 hours – for fever

CLOXACILLIN 500 mg 1 cap 4x a day for 7 days – antibiotic

AMBROXOL (MUCOSOLVAN) 75 mg 1 cap daily for 7 days – for cough

AZITHROMYCIN 500 mg 1 cap daily for 3 to 5 days

ADVICE:

Common cause of pneumonia is exposure to cold and non-treatment of ordinary upper respiratory tract infection like ordinary cough.

Chapter Four

Difficulty of Body Movement

FUNCTION LAETIA
(DIFFICULTY OF BODY MOVEMENT)

The objective of this chapter is to define which illness has greater hope of function return and where the cost of treatment may become a useless endeavor.

Function Laetia is the general term describing any difficulty of body movement, pain in movement, loss of movement and diminution of the capacity to move. There are several causes of this ailment and will be described in detail in the following pages. The reader must determine the specific area of dysfunction in order to know what the cause is.

Dysfunction of movement is not only caused by nerve impairment but also joint immobilization due to pain, physiologic problem, result of systemic illness and medication effect (anesthesia). Long term illness of malfunction may bring about permanent damage and loss of function of the affected part. Said ailment maybe become permanent and no amount of medication could bring back its function. Or, it may be temporary, of which, physiotherapy is a great help in bringing it back to function.

PARALYSIS

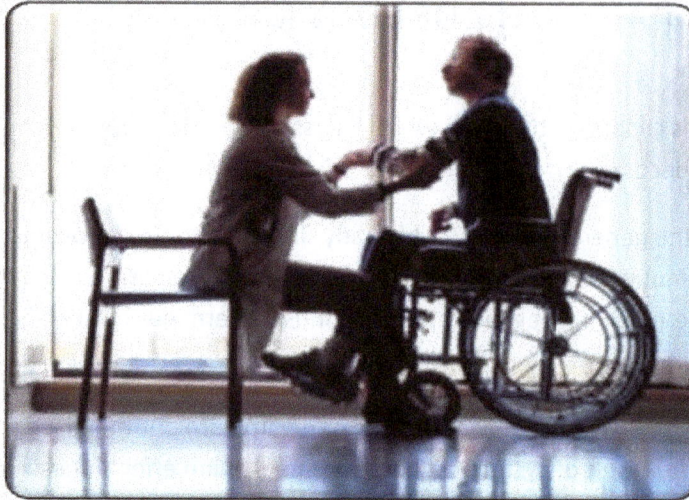

Hypertension is the main cause of paralysis. But there are other causes of paralysis of which the majority is caused by brain tumor and the rest due to trauma. Most paralysis does not revert to normal condition even with medication. But there are some successes. In stroke, for example, many have been brought back to productive capability with physiotherapy and long-term medications. The reader is then cautioned in pinning hope more than expected. The era of nerve regeneration is now a commonplace in western countries but still new and costly in the Philippines.

This chapter hopes to enlighten the reader the cause of paralysis and understand why and how the doctor manages his or her illness via medications and physiotherapy and what to expect. Hence, to understand why such laboratory examination and medication have to be taken for years and how to go about in the diagnostic examination is the main objective of this chapter.

PARALYSIS DUE TO STROKE

It is the loss of sensory and motor capability of a portion of the body due to HYPERTENSION.

DIAGNOSIS:

ORGAN INVOLVED: *brain*

CAUSE: rupture of brain blood vessel due to high blood pressure and the formation of a blood clot in the brain.

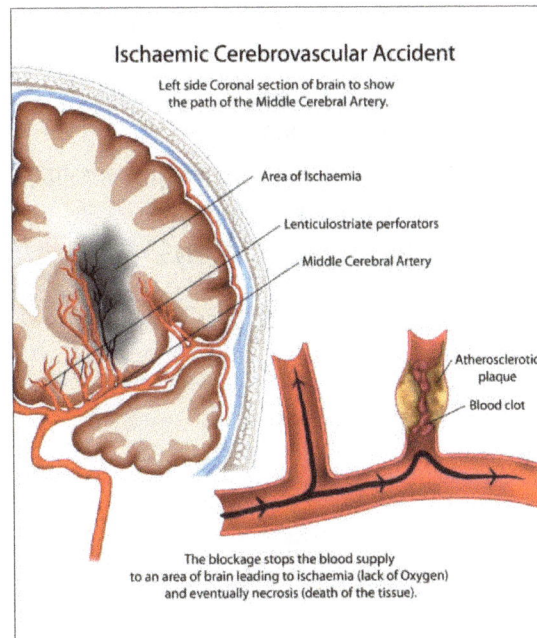

Ischaemic Cerebrovascular Accident

Left side Coronal section of brain to show the path of the Middle Cerebral Artery.

Area of Ischaemia

Lenticulostriate perforators

Middle Cerebral Artery

Atherosclerotic plaque

Blood clot

The blockage stops the blood supply to an area of brain leading to ischaemia (lack of Oxygen) and eventually necrosis (death of the tissue).

INITIAL TREATMENT:

METROPLOLOL 100 mh tablet daily

OR

NEFIDINE 10 mh tablet daily

CAPOTEN 25 mg tablet 2x a day

Elevate patient's head when lying down or upon collapse. Prevent aspiration if vomiting by turning head to the side. If convulsion is occurring, insert spoon inside the mouth

ADVICE:

Stroke is preventable. Daily monitoring of blood pressure and maintaining prescribed medicines are the only way to prevent stroke. The only time medications are stopped is when blood pressure goes down below 100/60 and they are not stopped if blood pressure is not known. Intake should not be based on what symptoms the patient feels for most of the time, they do not give the real blood pressure level. Some people do not feel any nuchal pain. Dizziness and heal fullness despite having high blood pressure.

LABORATORY EXAMINATIONS:

CT SCAN OF THE BRAIN – applied to determine the location of the blood clot and possible surgical removal.

DEFINITIVE TREATMENT: treatment is based on three stages
1. **CRANIOTOMY** – removal of the blood clot if it is massive and possible survival of the patient
2. **PHYSIOTHERAPY** – series of exercise to bring back function
3. **CONTINUATION OF ANTI – HYPERTENSIVE MEDICATIONS.**

PARALYSIS DUE TO TRAUMA TO THE HEAD

Paralysis secondary to vehicular accident, fall or mauling on the head.

DIAGNOSIS: CEREBRAL CONCUSSION / CEREBRAL HEMATOMA

ORGAN INVOLVED: *brain*

CAUSE: formation of a blood clot in the brain

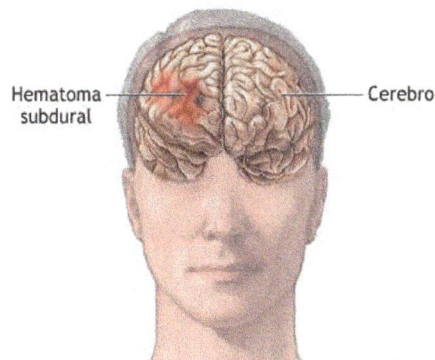

Hematoma subdural — Cerebro

INITIAL TREATMENT: none

ADVICE:

The survival of the patient is pinned on immediate diagnosis and treatment and the hospital is the only setting where these can be done.

LABORATORY EXAMINATIONS:

CT SCAN OF THE CRANIUM – no other modality is better than this diagnostic tool in locating the presence of blood in the brain.

DEFINITIVE TREATMENT:

CRANIOTOMY – the removal of the blood clot does not assure return of function

PARALYSIS DUE TO BRAIN TUMOR

Paralysis is usually preceded by chronic severe headaches, episodes of vomiting, loss of consciousness and the gradual loss of function of one side of the body, one limb of both upper and lower extremities on one side.

DIAGNOSE: BRAIN TUMOR

ORGAN INVOLVED: brain

CAUSE: TUMOR which maybe malignant or benign

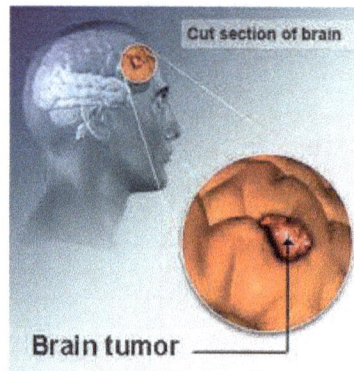

INITIAL TREATMENT

ANALGESICS: Mefenamic acid 550 mg tablet every 4 hours

ADVICE:

Tumors of the brain always manifest as headaches and often associated with other different symptoms all of which could be present in one person or they may not. The only hurdle one has to pass is to differentiate this illness from ordinary headaches such as migraine and eyestrain headaches. When vomiting accompanies these headaches, the possibility of brain tumor is high.

LABORATORY EXAMINATION:

CT SCAN OF THE CRANIUM – diagnose could only be attained through the use of this diagnostic tool. Location and the size of the tumor are definitely attained. The procedure is not intensive and traumatic to the patient involved. Planning for surgery could also be accomplished and the possibility of complete surgical removal could also be evaluated.

DEFINITIVE TREATMENT:

CRANIOTOMY – complete removal of the tumor is the objective of surgery. Malignancy limits the prognosis and of possible cure and is therefore of extreme importance to be taken into consideration when contemplating surgery. After surgery, the paralysis may persist and could not be alleviated. Therefore, this should be thoroughly discussed between the relatives and the surgeon in order to understand the outcome of the procedure.

PARALYSIS AFTER BACK BONE INJURY

Injury such as spinal fracture may result to paralysis of both upper and lower extremity (QUADRIPLEGIC) or paralysis of both lower limbs (PARAPLEGIC)

DIAGNOSIS: QUADRIPLEGIA OR PARAPLEGIA

ORGAN INVOLVED: spinal cord

CAUSE:

This is a severance of the spinal cord due to vertebral column fracture. Fracture of the vertebral column at the level of the neck may result to QUADRIPLEGIA. Fracture of the vertebral column at the level of the navel may result to PARAPLEGIA

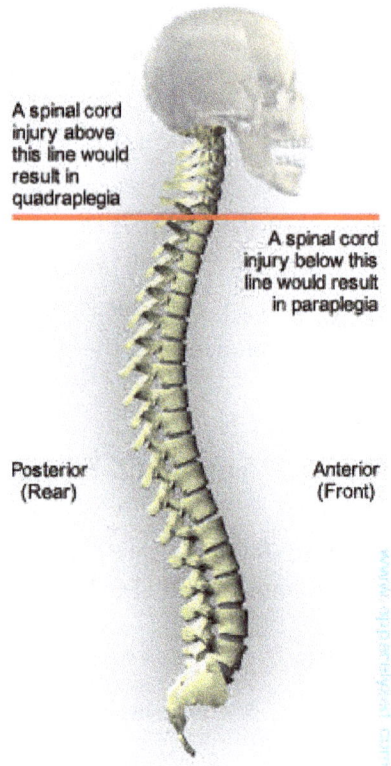

A spinal cord injury above this line would result in quadraplegia

A spinal cord injury below this line would result in paraplegia

Posterior (Rear)

Anterior (Front)

INITIAL TREATMENT:

STABILITY OF THE NECK INJURIES - when injured in an accident, the neck should be properly splinted or stabilized to prevent spinal cord severance. This could be accomplished by placing two heavy objects on each side of the head to prevent it from moving. Application of a broad plaster across the head would properly splint it. In the absence of a plaster, rope of any kind (or belt) should be used to tie the head down with the splint objects on each side of the head.

BACK INJURIES – prevention of severe torsion of the body of the injured in lifting or transferring. This is accomplished by placing the patient on a flat board such as a door in transporting the patient.

ADVICE:

QUADRIPLEGIA: If patients do not die in transport with injuries of the neck, they are more likely to end up with paralysis of the upper and lower extremities.

Patients whose injuries cause paralysis of both the upper and lower extremities may also cause paralysis of the breathing SYSTEMS (chest muscles and diaphragm). This complicates the management since the patient may need a ventilator – a machine that takes over the function of the lungs. This in turn will involve another surgery to make a temporary or permanent opening direct to the tubes of the lungs (BRONCHUS) which is done by making a TRACHEOSTOMY – an opening made at the front of the neck exposing the bronchus and an insertion of a curve tube where the ventilator is attached. Complications due to these ancillary procedures are so numerous to be written in detail. Patients may eventually die because of these complications.

PARAPLEGIA: Patient is paralyzed from abdomen down. Prognosis of this type of paralysis is much more positive. Care is directed towards bowel and urinary movement. If properly trained, the patient could do these on his own.

LABORATORY EXAMINATIONS:

X-RAY OF THE CERVICAL VERTEBRAE / LUMBROSCAL VERTEBRAE – x-rays done on the neck or back determine the extent of injury. It only shows the fractures where the involved vertebra is located. It does not show the extent of injury to spinal cord.

MAGNETIC RESONANCE IMAGING (MRI) – the complete examination of the spinal cord injury. It uses polarizing magnets to visualize any part of the body. Radiation is minimal compared to x-rays. 3D examination results are possible completely visualizing the extent of injury. With this modality, surgical planning can be completely done prior to intervention.

DEFINITIVE TREATMENT:

STABILIZATION OF THE SPINAL COLUMN - Currently, this is the only thing that medicine could do for this illness. Regeneration of the spinal cord is still in the experimental stage.

FRACTURES

Types of Fractures

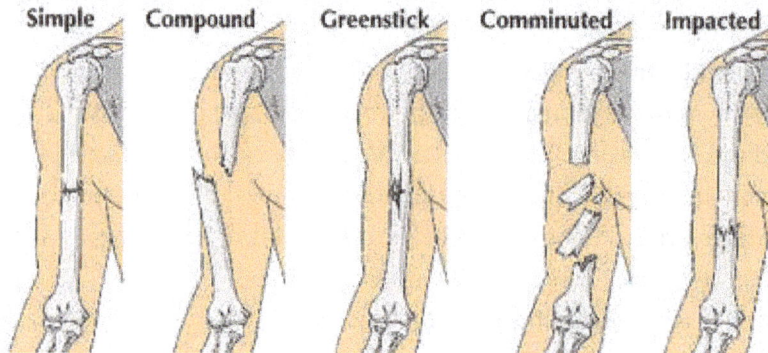

Simple · Compound · Greenstick · Comminuted · Impacted

The initial symptom that a person feels when a fracture occurs in any bone of the body is dysfunction of the affected part: limitation of the movement (Function Laetia) and pain on movement. If bleeding occurs near the fracture itself, hematoma or blackening of the surrounding tissue follows. In the presence of these two signs, the necessity of doing x-rays is a must.

Fracture of any part of the body necessitates splinting to prevent further injury to the nearby tissues. On the extremities, this can be accomplished by placing of wood at the side of the fractured area trying both ends with a piece of cloth to the affected limb. The use of elastic bandages is the most appropriate but in the absence of these, long strips of cloth would suffice.

In the absence of open wounds, most fractures in the young can be treated by plaster casts. This is usually in place for the next 3 months and follow up x-rays are done to determine fracture healing. Loosening of the plaster cast is an indication for recasting if the fracture is not yet healed.

Open wounds in fractures necessitate debridement by surgery and application of bone stabilizers such as: INTRAMEDULLARY NAIL, external fixators, screws, wires and plates. These devices are usually removed after fracture healing but some surgeons prefer them to be in place for life.

Chapter Five

Difficulty of Breathing

DIFFICULTY OF BREATHING

The objective of the schematic diagram in the following pages is to provide a clear understanding of the causes, as well as, the organs involved. By following through the diagram, the reader is then led to specific treatments.

The medical term for difficulty of breathing is DYSPNEA. And this is due to varied reasons from the simplest cause (overweight) to the most complicated illness (CHRONIC OBSTRUCTIVE PULMONARY DISEASE). This illness also involves different organ system and different etiologies. Discussing them one by one would cause confusion to the layman. What is important for the reader is for him to understand what the cause of his difficulty of breathing is, know the emergency treatment, decide which specialty he or she has to go to and to understand fully what his doctor recommends. This chapter only presents the most common illness and does not attempt to cover all lung diseases.

DIFFICULTY OF BREATHING

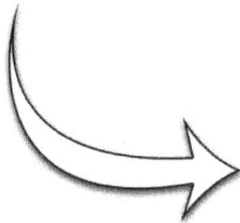

TO INHALE:
Breathing movement is impeded or restricted and in seemed to flow down to the middle of the chest only. A history of productive cough(phlegm yellowish). fever and chest pains of not more than ywo weeks cough is noted to produce gurgling sound inside the chest

DIAGNOSE:
ACUTE PNEUMONIA

ORGAN INVOLED:
LUNGS

CAUSE:
BACTERIAL

LAB EXAM:
CHEST X-RAYS

TREATMENT:
TEQUIN 400mg 1 tab daily for 7 days

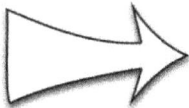

TO INHALE & EXHALE:
Breathingis limited to both inhilation and exhalation. in either way no amount os air is adequate for the patient. He usually has history of smoking or chronic lungdisease such as TB.

DIAGNOSIS:
CHRONIC OBSTRUCTIVE PULMONARY DISEASE

ORGAN INVOLVED:
LUNGS

CAUSE:
Destruction of alveoli in the lubngs

LAB EXAM:
Pulmonary function test

TREATMENT:
SPIRIVA inhiation capsules daily

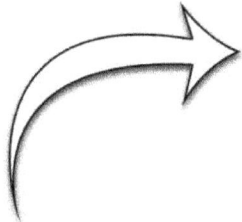

TO EXHALE:
Bring out air is limited and rstricted. This is often chronic and last for years occuring on and off and triggered by cold climate, dust, anxiety and chemicals. Cough is dry or it may be productive of white phlegm.

DIAGNOSIS:
BRONCHIAL ASTHMA

ORGAN INVOLVED:
LUNGS

CAUSE:
Hereditary

LAB EXAM:
skin testing for allergy

TREATMENT:
SALBUTAMOL 1 tab 3x a day

DIFFICULTY OF BREATHING

ON EXERTION:
Climbing stairs or walking short distance trigger difficulty of breathing.

DIAGNOSE:
CONGESTIVE HEART FAILURE

ORGAN INVOLED:
HEART

CAUSE:
HEART FAILURE

LAB EXAM:
ECG

TREATMENT:
LANOXIN 1 tab 3x a day

JUST SITTING DOWN:
Small, frequent gasps of air, non restricted asso with bloating of the face and swelling of the feet

DIAGNOSIS:
UREMIA

ORGAN INVOLVED:
KIDNEY

CAUSE:
KIDNEY FAILURE

LAB EXAM:
CREATININE

TREATMENT:
DIALYSIS

UPON PLAYING:
Patient suddenly stops and sit, becomes pale and gasps for air for a few minutes. He goes back playing after a while.

DIAGNOSIS:
ASTRIAL SEPTAL DEFECT

ORGAN INVOLVED:
HEART

CAUSE:
Failure to close in the womb

LAB EXAM:
2D ECHO

TREATMENT:
SURGERY

DIFFICULTY OF BREATHING DUE TO STAB WOUND, FRACTURE OF RIBS … see stab wounds of the chest.

221

Chapter Six

CYSTS AND CANCER

CYSTS AND CANCER

All cancers in any part of the body show as a tumor or new growth. But not all cysts or new growth is cancerous or will evolve to cancer. Only a fraction of them are cancer. Current findings show that cancerous tumors start as cancer from the beginning. The evolution of a non – cancerous tumor to a cancerous one is very rare. No vitamin or health style could prevent cancer from forming. Thus, no treatment whatsoever could cure cancer. Present medical treatments are geared towards prolonging life for a few years and never aimed to cure anyone from cancer. If anyone is claiming otherwise, either he is fooling someone or is selling something for business sake.

No laboratory exam could match the accuracy of a biopsy to diagnose cancer. Mammography, CT-scans, ultrasound findings and x-rays results are probable diagnoses but they are not specific diagnosis to rely on, in managing a cancer. They only serve as working diagnosis in order to find the real etiology of a tumor. Therefore, all are probabilities until a biopsy is done and a histopathologic finding confirms the diagnosis of cancer.

Some of the associated signs and symptoms of cancer in any part of the body are LOSS OF WEIGHT and PAIN in the location where the tumor is. When these two general symptoms appear, most of the time, the cancer is in its late stage. Prognosis or predicting the outcome of a cancer is based on the spread of cancer. The further the spread of the cancer, the shorter the life span of the patient. The bigger the primary tumor (the first new growth) when found, the shorter the life span of the patient. Thus, the smaller the primary tumor is found, the better for the patient. This is where annual physical examination and general checkup come in. A layman may find a new growth as nothing but it could be the beginning of a cancerous tumor. ***Immediate biopsy upon discovery is the dictum in fighting cancer.***

BREAST CYSTS AND CANCER

Most cysts in the breast are not cancer. Only 5% of those cysts found in the breast are cancer. Awareness of a cyst in the breast by a woman no matter the age, is stepping stone in the fight against cancer. Cancerous tumors found less than 2 cm will increase the life span of a woman fourfold. Some women would even have normal life span when these tumors are removed immediately. Thus, BIOPSY is your best option in the fight against breast cancer. Mammography only identifies a probable presence of a tumor. No more, no less. It cannot make a diagnosis of cancer. It is not 100% accurate in identifying whether a tumor is malignant or not – the most important factor in the management of cancer. It may lead the physician to recommend biopsy since it can mark a new growth of less than 1 cm - a tumor size that no surgeon could feel upon examination of the breast.

There are three ways to do BIOPSY:

1. **FINE NEEDLE BIOPSY -** wherein a syringe with a big needle is injected on the exact site of the breast tumor (with anesthesia) and forceful aspiration of a tumor tissue is done. This in turn is brought to the laboratory for examination (HISTOPHATOLOGIC EXAMINATION – histopath). The setback with this method is that the patient is left with the tumor if it is found out to be benign. She has no recourse but to undergo A SECOND SUGERY for total excision. No patient would like to live with a tumor remaining in her breast. On the other hand, if the tumor is found to be a cancer, the method is not traumatic to the patient since no surgery was done on her person in the first visit.

2. **EXCISIONAL BIOPSY -** A small opening is made on the breast under local anesthesia and the whole or part of the tumor (if it is too large for a minor surgery) is removed. This is brought to the laboratory for HISTOPATH. The advantage of doing this technique is the complete removal of the tumor, assuring the patient of totality (with benign tumors). But when the tumor is discovered to be cancer, the thought of undergoing another surgery is a convincing obstacle to the doctor.

3. **DOUBLE SET UP WITH FROZEN SECTION –** This is done by doing the biopsy inside the main operating theater and prepared to do the major surgery. A small incision is initially done on the breast under local anesthesia or general anesthesia, whichever, the patient prefers. (Local anesthesia allows the patient to discuss with the surgeon the outcome of the initial biopsy and decide). A portion of the mass or the entire tumor is removed and brought to the laboratory. Pathologists freeze and a preliminary reading is done. This entails a larger expense, since the pathologist is asked to stand by and wait until the specimen is brought to him. Examination of the specimen is hurriedly done, and more often than not, the size of the specimen may not be adequate to arrive into a definitive diagnosis. Some patients may not be in their proper perspective to decide right there and then, and therefore, a major surgery that

will affect her whole life. On the other hand, the patient is not left hanging for several anxious days waiting for the result of the biopsy.

Symptoms of advanced or late stage breast cancers:
1. Swelling and reddening of a part or the entire breast
2. Ulceration (wound) or pus formation
3. Orange peeling of the skin (skin of the breast appear like orange peel with dimpling of the hair follicles)
4. Hardening of the skin like tanned leather
5. Darkening of the skin like eggplant

CHEST PAIN in these instances, radiotherapy is done first prior to removal of the entire breast followed by chemotherapy. In the advent of so many techniques in the management of breast cancer, it has led to different protocols. Upon diagnosis of breast cancer through biopsy, the two current major ones are:

1. MODIFIED RADICAL MASTECTOMY – Removal of the entire breast leaving the muscles beneath it. And removal of all lymph nodes and cleaning the area under the muscles and below the clavicle. If the primary tumor size is less than 2 cm and there are no positive lymph nodes (to cancer), NO CHEMOTHERAPY, NO RADIOTHERAPY.
   - If the primary tumor size is less than 2cm but there are positive lymph nodes even a single one, patient is advised to have chemotherapy.
   - If the primary tumor size is more than 2 cm even without positive (with cancer cells) lymph node, chemotherapy as advised.
2. Removal of the entire tumor and surrounding tissues up to 1 cm (LUMPECTOMY) only leaving the rest of the breast in its entirely (shape, size, counter). It is followed by chemotherapy and radiotherapy

Studies have shown that two different modalities have the same outcome in the aspect of survival rate. But the quality of life, short recovery, short hospital stay, surgical complications and psychological impact are better with the second option.

TUMORS AND CANCERS OF THE INTESTINE

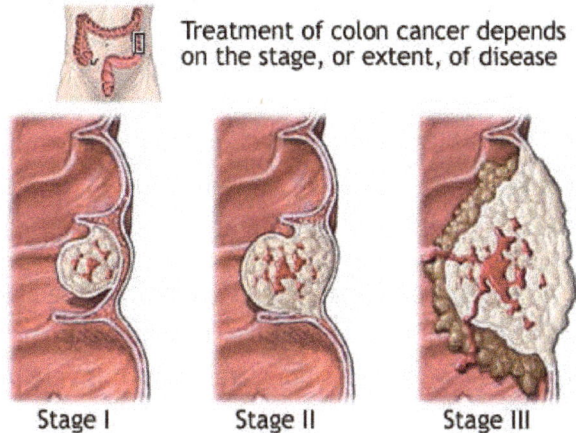

Treatment of colon cancer depends on the stage, or extent, of disease

Stage I   Stage II   Stage III

Symptoms of tumors and cancers of the GASTROINTESTINAL TRACT depend on the location. But the general symptoms a person will feel when a tumor is present are:

1. BLOATEDNESS – food and the intestinal content cannot pass through the obstruction caused by the tumor.
2. BLOOD is present in the stools – It may present as blackening of the stool of frank fresh blood depending on the location of the tumor. If it is farther up (stomach), it may show as tarry stools or dark streaks in the stools. If it is way down (anus), fresh blood may accompany the stools.
3. PAIN – It is not specific. Abdominal pain may be relieved by medications or it may not. Bowel movement may trigger pain or it may relieve it. It may be colicky or gnawing. And no specific location of the abdomen may pin point which part of the intestine is involved.

If the tumor or cancer is in the **esophagus**, a person may feel pain on the chest and difficulty of swallowing solid food.

If the tumor is located in the **stomach and small intestines,** early satiety, pain upon food intake, crampy abdominal pain, vomiting is among the symptoms that often manifest.

If the tumor is located in the **large intestines,** constipation or alternate watery stool and constipation may occur. Abdominal pain and fresh blood may be present.

Diagnosis can be attained by X-RAY or ENDOSCOPY:

X-RAYS:

UPPER GI SERIES – with the patient on NPO (nothing per orem) from midnight to hour of examination, he is asked to swallow a milk – like substance and x – rays are taken. This will visualize the esophagus down to the small intestine.

BARIUM ENEMA – Cleansing of the large intestine is done the night before by enema. Then, a catheter is inserted through the anus and milk – like substance is pumped in to the intestines. The patient is asked to hold it until all x – rays positions are taken. It is very uncomfortable and may not be good for the elderly.

ENDOSCOPY:

GASTROSCOPY – it is the insertion of a fiber – optic tube the size of small finger into the mouth down to the stomach and duodenum. The inside of the stomach can be seen through a TV monitor or direct through the instrument. The advantage of this method is the capacity to biopsy the tumor immediately.

COLONOSCOPY – after a cleansing enema, a fiber – optic tube is inserted through the anus and the large intestines can be visualized. Biopsy can be done at the same time or the entire tumor if it is small can be removed in situ.

Treatment of benign tumors is total excision. Cancer in the Gastro – intestinal tract consists mainly of resection or removal of the affected portion by surgery.

ESOPHAGECTOMY – removal of the esophagus

GASTRECTOMY – resection of the stomach

HEMICOLECTOMY – is the removal of a portion of the large intestine.

TOTAL COLECTOMY – removal of the entire large intestine

MILES RESECTION – is the removal of a portion of the large intestine including the anus. In this surgery, the intestine is diverted and attached to the side of the abdomen creating a COLOSTOMY, where the patient would then pass his stools permanently. This surgery is indicated when the cancer involves a portion of the large intestine so near the anus.

The continuity of the GASTROINTESTINAL TRACT is managed by several ways:

1. END TO END ANASTOMOSIS – remaining portion of the intestine is attached to each other. This is done when the segments are proximal to each other and no tension is created upon attachment.
2. END TO SIDE ANASTOMOSIS – approximation of segments creates disparity if intestinal lumen size. So, attachment is made with one end sutured to the side of other portion of the intestine.
3. TRANSPOSITION OF AN INTESTINAL SEGMENT – a distal part of the GASTROINESTINAL TRACT is resected and transposed to the area of surgery where ends do not meet. A segment of the small intestine or a part of the large intestine is often employed in this maneuver.
4. CREATION OF AN INTESTINAL TUBE – a portion of the stomach is fashioned to make a tube – like structure. This is often used in the reconstruction of the esophagus.

Chemotherapy and radiotherapy only improve survival rate about 3 to 4 years. If the cancer is resected at an early stage (before spread to other parts of the body – metastasis), survival rate is longer. If diagnosed at a later stage, prognosis is poor and the patient will only last for 6 months.

TUMORS OF THE LIVER

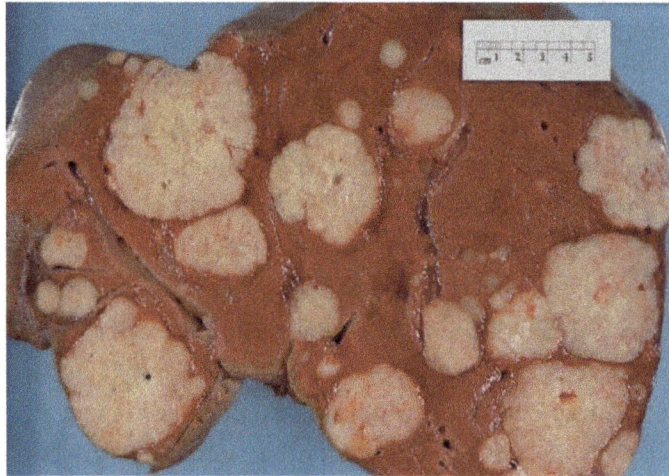

There are benign tumors of the liver that would exist without affecting the patient. They are generally termed as HEPATIC CYSTS. Some of them may be due to intake of medications (ESTROGEN INTAKE), infectious diseases (AMOEBIC ABSCESS), and hereditary (BENIGN HEPATIC CYST). No treatment is required except for those which are in infectious in origin. They may be found on general physical examination and routine laboratory examinations and may cause so much anxiety to the patient. Assurance and diagnostic biopsy are the only tools required to obtain peace of mind.

Recent findings show that CANCER OF THE LIVER may have evolved from HEPATITIS B infection, AMOEBIC COLITIS and subsequent AMOEBIC ABSCESS, chemical exposure, radiation and heredity. But there is no absolute cause and effect finding. Not all sufferers (patients who developed) of Hepatitis B develop cancer of the liver and not all cancer of the liver had Hepatitis B in their history. Like all the other cancers, medicine is not absolutely certain about its origin.

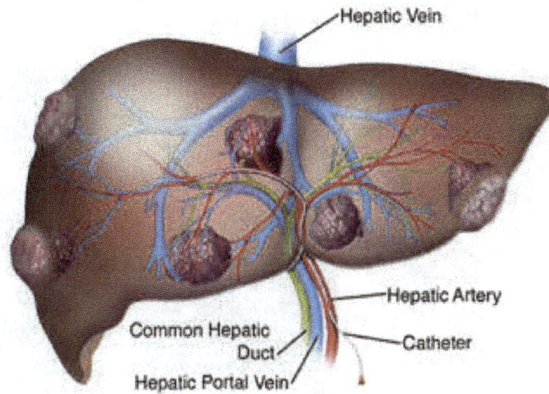

LABORATORY EXAMINATIONS:

ULTRASOUND OF THE LIVER – tumors of the liver of any kind can be detected by this method. But it does not classify which is cancerous and which is benign.

ALPHAFETO PROTEIN – is a blood examination that could detect cancer of the liver 95% of the time. This is often used to determine the etiology of a tumor found on routine ultrasound of the liver.

FINE NEEDLE BIOPSY – a long needle is inserted into the right upper quadrant of the abdomen (RUQ) direct to the liver and a sample is aspirated and brought to the laboratory. This is the definitive diagnostic exam to classify which tumor is malignant or benign.

CT SCAN OF THE LIVER – this is done to determine the possibility of surgical removal of the tumor.

DEFINITIVE TREATMENT:

HEPATIC LOBECTOMY – a lobe of the liver is totally removed. This is only indicated if the cancer is confined to one lobe. Presence of metastasis (spread) does not warrant this operation.

TOTAL HEPATECTOMY – total removal of the liver. This is followed by liver transplant. Most of these operations are a failure and are considered to be experimental because of frequent rejection of the donor liver.

Chemotherapy and radiotherapy are failures in prolonging survival.

CANCER OF THE LUNGS

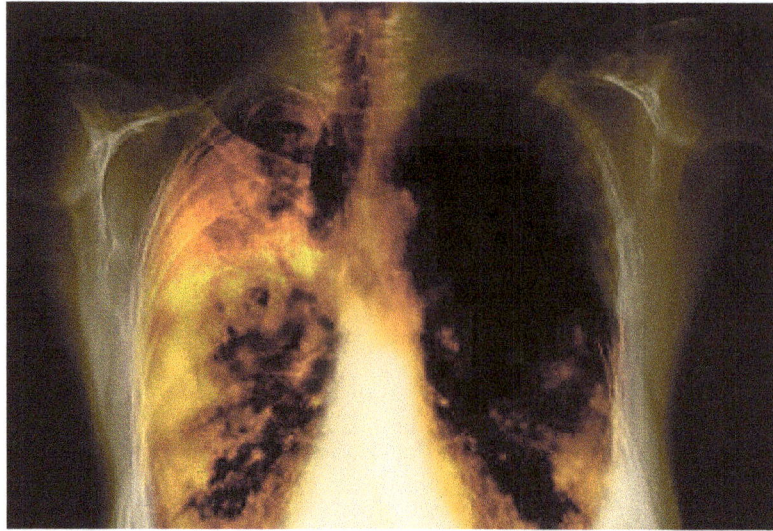

Smoking is the main cause of cancer of the lungs. There are other factors that may contribute to the cause but are only probabilities due to the absence of cause and effect gradients.

Patients who develop cancer of the lungs start as pain in the back or chest. Mark loss of weight and blood in the sputum follow after several weeks. This is often mistaken for tuberculosis and is often the cause for the misdiagnosis.

Chest x-ray is the diagnostic exam that detects the lesion. It may show lesions that are not pathognomonic of cancer and could be mistaken for something else.

CT SCAN guided fine needle biopsy definitely attains (the required) diagnosis.

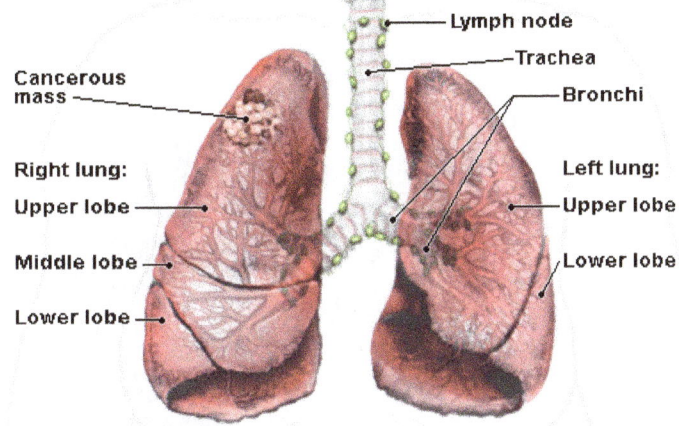

Lung Cancer

Lymph node — Trachea — Bronchi

Cancerous mass

Right lung:
Upper lobe
Middle lobe
Lower lobe

Left lung:
Upper lobe
Lower lobe

Early diagnosis has never been attained. When diagnosed patients only have a few months to live despite any kind of treatment modality which include:

PULMONARY LOBECTOMY – it is the removal of one lobe of the lungs.

TOTAL PULMONARY LOBECTOMY – total removal of one side of the lungs.

Alternative medicines have claimed to improve survival rate. To this date, no scientific data has backed this claim.

TUMORS OF THE UTERUS

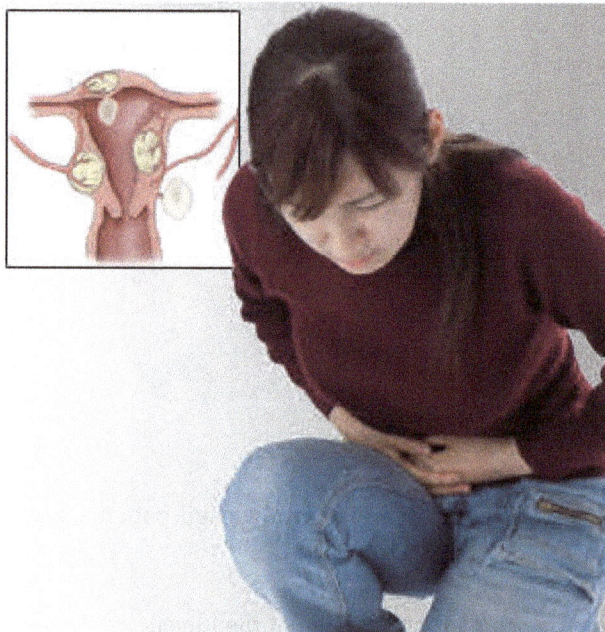

Tumors of the uterus and its adnexa are often missed on physical examination. When they are less than 2 cm, the palpating fingers of the doctor could not feel the tumors that are often covered by the presence of the intestine above it, the urinary bladder and the position of the uterus, thus, symptoms that the patient feel would lead to their presence.

Vaginal spotting, profuse menstruations and irregular menstruation are the main symptoms of uterine tumors. Any irregularity of the menstrual period should alert the patient of a possible presence of a mass or a tumor.

Pain is another symptom that often accompanies tumors in the uterus. This is often associated with the menstrual period and becomes more severe as the tumor enlarges.

Some patients may have enlargement of the abdomen that is often mistaken for pregnancy. Watchful review of the menstrual days should alert a woman whether she is really pregnant or not.

Myoma is the most common benign tumor of the uterus. Indication for removal of the entire uterus includes massive vaginal bleeding and necrosis of the myoma. Tumors can arise from the ovary, fallopian tube, uterus and cervix. Differentiation of these tumors from the malignant ones is the most important factor in the diagnostic procedure.

Cancer could arise from any part of the uterus and adnexae. Early diagnosis is the main objective in the management of said disease. Biopsy of the tumor is the only definitive diagnostic exam that could differentiate benign tumors from malignant.

LABORATORY EXAMINATIONS:

ULTRASOUND OF THE UTERUS AND ADNEXAE – the cheapest way to diagnose any tumor in the uterus. This can be done   Trans – vaginal (probe is inserted into the vagina) or Trans abdominal (above the abdomen).

PAPS SMEAR – routine diagnostic exam to determine any cancer of the cervix and uterus. This is done by scraping the surface of the cervix with a wooden spatula

DEFINITVE TREATMENT:

TOTAL ABDOMINAL HYSTERECTOMY – OOPHORECTOMY (TABHSO) - is the removal of the entire uterus including the ovaries and fallopian tubes. This can be done through vagina (TRANSVAGINAL TABHSO) or by opening the abdomen. (TRANSABDOMINAL TABHSO)

HYSTERECTOMY – removal of the uterus alone spares the ovaries.

TUMOR OF THE BRAIN

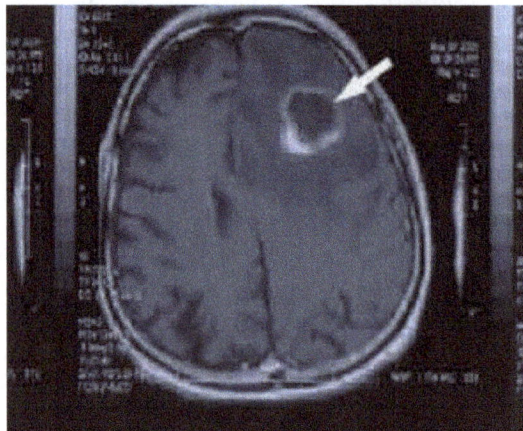

Tumors of the brain whether it is benign or malignant have the same manifestation. Primary symptom often felt is severe headache. Other signs and symptoms depend on where the location of the tumor is. If the visual center of the brain is affected, visual problems are usually suffered by the patient; if the motor center of the brain is affected, paralysis is noted on one side of the patient. If the talk center is affected, the patient will lose his capacity to speak. Distinguishing ordinary headaches from headaches due to brain tumors is one difficult hurdle to make. Some patients may carry the brain tumor without much symptom. But others may have severe migraine headaches. As the tumor enlarges, signs of weakness and even complete paralysis affect the contra – lateral side: if the tumor is on the left side of the brain, the paralyzed portion of the body is on the left side (arms and legs); if the tumor is in the left side of the brain, the affected part is on the right side. Severity of headache and paralysis, by themselves, cannot make one distinguish between benign from cancerous tumors. Only by biopsy could one distinguish between the two. And it is only through CT SCAN could a diagnosis be attained. Ordinary x-rays and ultrasound do not accomplish this.

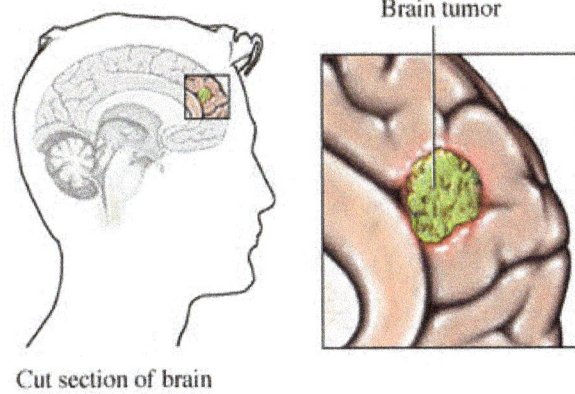

Brain tumor

Cut section of brain

With the advent of precision laser surgery, removal of tumors in the brain has greatly improved. Mortality rate has gone down but the expense has gone up.

CANCER OF THE THROAT

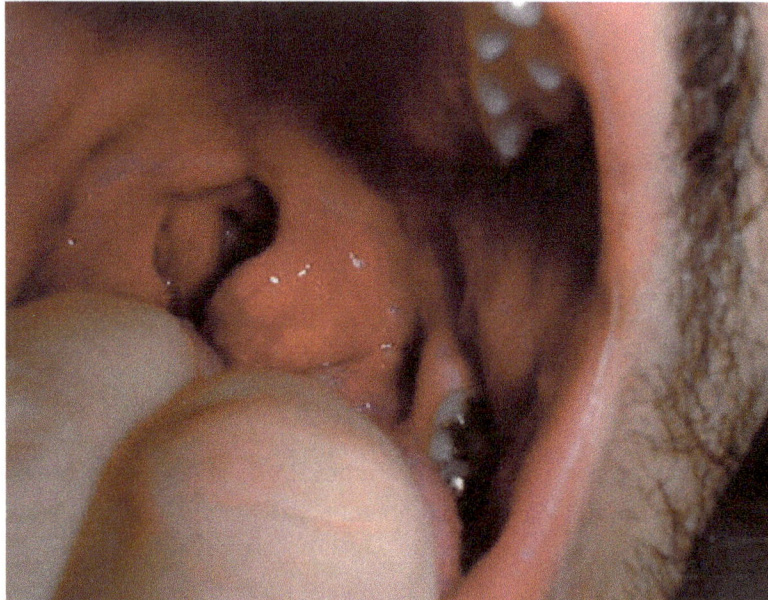

The disease can affect different parts of the throat.

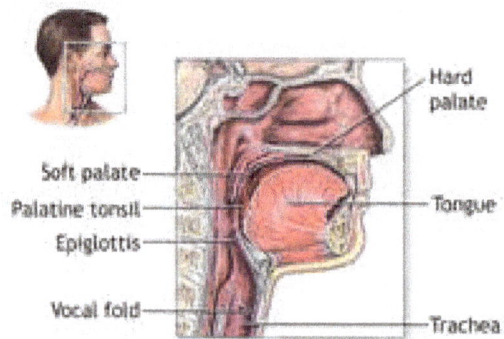

It may affect the larynx and so the symptoms often manifest as long standing hoarseness. It may affect the first portion of the esophagus and could start as difficulty of swallowing. It may affect the pharynx (back side of the throat) and would manifest as sore throat that do not heal with any antibiotics. Individuals mostly affected by this disease come from the ethnic Chinese groups, the reasons of which, no one knows. Diagnosis is accomplished by biopsy of the mass found in these are aided by CT scan or direct visualization. Treatment is complete surgical removal of the tumor and surrounding tissues plus denudation or cleaning of the neck on the side of the tumor. Prognosis is poor and many patients do not respond to chemotherapy or radiotherapy to warrant a good 5 years survival.

CYSTS AND CANCER OF THE SKIN

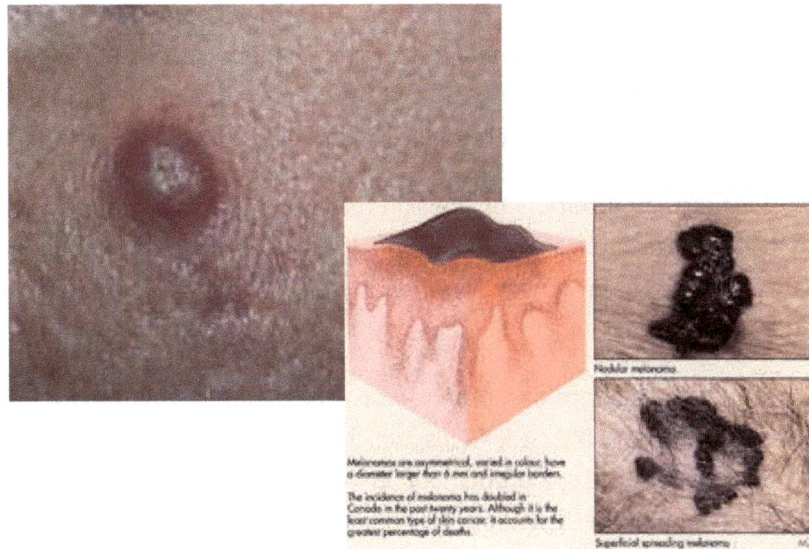

There are many new growths of the skin that are considered as benign. Most of them are in the category of INCLUSION CYSTS or cysts due to obstruction of a normal sweat function among them are:

SEBACEOUS CYST – cyst form in the obstruction of the skin pores of the sweat gland usually due to dirt or old skin. It incorporates a fine whitish and odorous material usually concentrates of sweat elements.

Though benign, these tumors enlarge to tremendous sizes and may become infected. In diabetics, this is the precursor of large ulcerations of the skin requiring extensive treatment including skin grafting. When infected, the difficulty of removing the entire cyst including the sac warrants initial incision and drainage followed by excision of the cyst proper. Due to this, when found, sebaceous cyst should be removed immediately no matter the size or location. Careful dissection of the entire sac should be done to prevent recurrence.

EPIDERMOID CYST – It is an inclusion cyst that is found underneath the skin which may or may not be sweat gland in origin. This is harder in consistency than the sebaceous cyst and slow in growth. If the location of the cyst is found over nerve terminals, it may elicit pain or numbness.

LIPOMA – yellowish fatty ovoid mass found under the skin, which may not manifest any symptom. Indication for surgery is usually cosmetic and the fear of cancer development; unfounded since this tumor do not progress into cancer. But differentiation of lipoma from lymphomatous tumor is necessary since their appearance is markedly the same. Location of the tumor may give the differential diagnosis since lymphomatous tumors, which have cancerous tendencies, are often found under the axilla.

PAPILLOMA – pedunculated tumors of the skin (hanging on a stalk) are benign but they grow into large sizes (fist of a child). They are very vascular and thus bleed profusely when lacerated. Excision is necessary for cosmetic reasons. These tumors are often found in areas that impede movement and are ugly in appearance.

GANGLION CYST – cysts that are found on top or near ligaments and tendons such as in the wrists and popliteal area. They contain jellylike clear fluids, which easily burst on puncture. When left on its own, the tumor does not enlarge nor cause symptoms. But some cysts may cause limitation of movement in the wrist and pain in the popliteal (back of the knee). The usual indication for surgery is pain and cosmetics.

FUNICULITIS – an inflammatory reaction of the sub – epidermal layer of the skin (layer of skin below surface). Cause is unknown but has connection with SKIN TUBERCULOSIS, SKIN ASTHMA and all kinds of allergies. These cysts are tiny; sometimes the size of ball – points of ball pens, hard and moves when felt and are not tender or painful. Surgery is not necessary and is often tedious to do. Antibiotics do not have any effect and are not part of the management.

SKIN TAGS – skin extensions which do not contain anything. They exist in cluster and are often found in the axilla. They are associated with VON RECKLINGHAUSENS' DISEASE but no significant mortality or morbidity could be found.

MOLE – pigmented inclusion cyst that may or may not progress into a cancerous tumor. Biopsy is necessary with moles which pigmentation extends farther from the base including the surrounding skin.

Cancer of the skin is classified into:

1. **MELANOMA** – a skin hyper – pigmentation (darkening of the skin) usually found in the sun – exposed portions of the body. Caucasians rather than the colored people are affected by this cancer. Biopsy is the only method of diagnosis. Wide excision is usually adequate to remove the cancer at an early stage. But if left unmanaged, this may spread to the liver, lungs and brain.
2. **SQUAMOUS CANCER** – cancer found near the mouth, nose, and anus. This usually arises from the smooth surface of these areas and enlarges to a large size and ulcerates emitting foul odor. When found, wide excision is necessary to stop spread of the cancer. Chemotherapy and radiotherapy may help in extending the life of the patient.
3. **BASAL CELL CARCINOMA** – arise from areas with abundant sweat glands. They may not spread to other parts of the body but they destroy structures near or under them. They progress into big ulcerations with foul smelling discharges. Wide excision is the treatment of choice.

ENLARGEMENT OF THE NECK

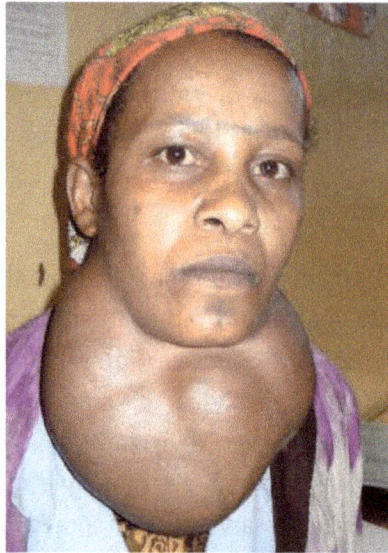

Enlargement of the neck associated with bulging of the eyes, palpitation, irritability, loss of weight despite good appetite, dry skin, intolerance to heat or cold

DIAGNOSIS: TOXIC GOITER

CAUSE: Iodine deficiency

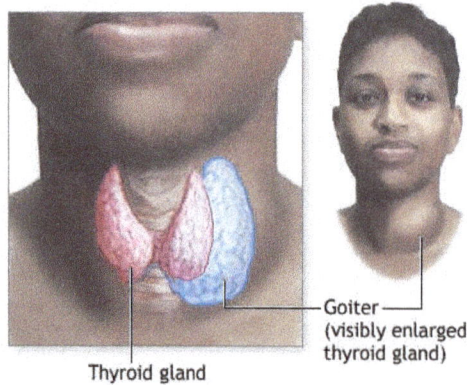

Thyroid gland

Goiter
(visibly enlarged
thyroid gland)

241

ORGAN INVOLVED: *thyroid*

INITIAL TREATMENT: none

ADVICE:

Enlargement of the neck due to TOXIC GOITER is always accompanied by the symptoms mentioned above. When these symptoms are absent, the disease is still TOXIC GOITER but in the EUTHYROID STATE. This illness has to be differentiated from other illnesses presenting as enlargement of the neck such as THYROID ADENOMA.

Which is a cyst formation of the organ THYROID; THYROID CANCER
This is enlargement of the neck but spreads fast to other organs of the body. This difference is in the hands of the doctor with his use of laboratory.

LABORATORY EXAMINATIONS:

T3 – T4 – examination of the blood taken anytime even without fasting to determine the level of the hormone THYROXINE – a hormone produced by the THYROID used by the body for energy. An increase indicates TOXIC GOITER. A normal level of THYROXINE indicates EUTHYROID STATE of a GOITER DISEASE. A low level of THYROXINE indicates HYPOTHYROID state of a GOITER DISEASE.

THYROID STIMULATING HORMONE (TSH) determination - hormone produced by the pituitary an organ below the brain, responsible for stimulating the THYROID to produce its own hormone THYROXIN. This usually decreases in time of TOXIC GOITER, during treatment and increase after removal of the thyroid in surgery.

ULTRASOUND OF THE ANTERIOR NECK – Ultrasound done on the neck to determine the cause of the enlargement. This differentiates solid enlargement from cysts formation (liquid containing) inside the thyroid.

RADIOACTIVE IODINE UPTAKE (RAIU) – it is an injection of a radioactive drug or tablet taken before the day of the x-ray like procedure. Scan is done in front of the neck to determine the uptake of the drug into the thyroid. Any increase of the radioactive material inside the THYROID indicates TOXIC GOITER (shown in the x-ray film as darkening of a part). Absence of the radioactive material inside the THYROID indicates malignancy or cystic formation (liquid type of tumor). This is labeled by the RADIOLOGIST as HOT (when the radioactive material is taken up by the thyroid) or COLD (when the radioactive material is not taken up by the thyroid).

DEFINITVE TREATMENT:

IODINE TABLET – A tablet once a day to be taken for 2 years. There is usually noted a hardening of thyroid and gradual decrease of the enlargement of the neck. But some do not respond to this method of treatment even with prolonged medication.

THIAMAZOLE 30 mg tablet daily for 3 months or until the level of the T3 – T4 determination goes down to normal level.

PROPRANOLOL 10 mh tablet 3x a day. This drug is used to control the symptoms of irritability, palpitation, nervousness, etc. and is usually taken until a symptom of TOXIC GOITER abates.

RADIO ACTIVE IODINE INJECTION – A radioactive iodinated medicine is injected into the veins to burn the THYROID and stop its hyper-function. This is usually given to older persons above 40 years rather than to young individuals because it may cause HYPOTHYROIDISM. This is also used to burn the remaining tissues of a cancerous tumor in the thyroid.

THYROIDECTOMY – Surgical removal of the thyroid which could be partial or total depending on the size of the enlargement. More often than not, this is resorted to by the patients themselves for cosmetic reasons. Complications include loss of voice, hoarseness and loss of high in singing. In good hands, all of these complications do not happen IF TOTAL THYDROIDECTOMY is done, HYPOTHYDROIDISM may occur and thus, lifelong intake of THYROID hormone is a must. Symptoms of HYPOTHYROIDISM include generalized weakness, swelling and edema of the entire body, cramps and retraction of the tongue causing asphyxia. HYPOPARATHYROIDISM may also occur due to the inadvertent removal of the parathyroid gland located at the back of the THYROID. Patients suffer tetany and cramps due to the loss of calcium.

MASS IN THE ANTERIOR NECK

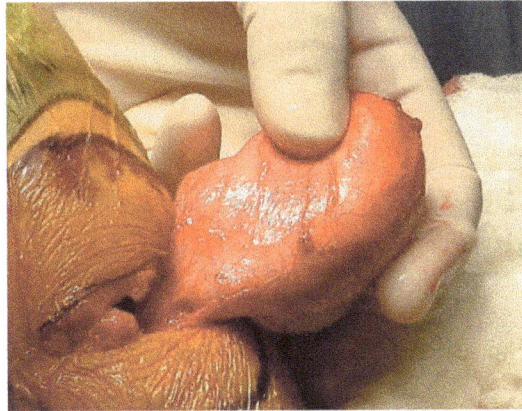

It is a tumor or cyst that is forming at the front of the neck without any other signs and symptoms which gradually enlarges without pain. This is often noticed by other people rather than by the patients themselves.

DIAGNOSIS: THYROID TUMOR which could be benign or malignant

ORGAN INVOLVED: *thyroid*

CAUSE: unknown. It forms inside the thyroid and gradually enlarges.

INITIAL TREATMENT: none

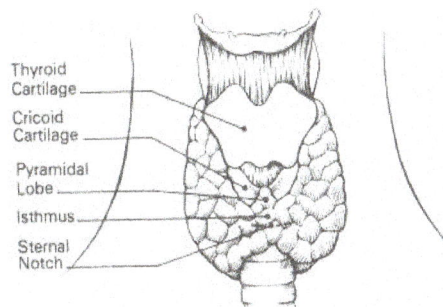

ADVICE:

When a mass or tumor is noticed in the neck, this should be brought to physician to determine the cause. The importance of medical consultation is emphasized because a lot of malignant tumors start as an ordinary lump and gradually enlarged to a size that disturbs swallowing of food. It is only through laboratory examinations that tumors can be differentiated.

LABORATORY EXAMINATIONS:

ULTRASOUND OF THE ANTERIOR NECK – By sound waves, tumor in the neck can be differentiated whether it is made up of liquid or solid.

FINE NEEDLE BIOPSY – A large needle is injected into the mass in the neck and forcefully aspirated. Small tissues of the tumor is taken and brought to the laboratory. This will determine whether the mass is malignant or benign (not cancer).

THYROID SCAN – A radioactive iodine tablet is taken before the day of the examination. Then, the patient is brought inside a machine that will scan his neck. Concentration of the radioactive iodine in any part of the tumor will show as hyperactivity or HOT NODULE signifying benign (not cancer) in many cases. Cold nodules may mean cancerous tumor. But this examination is not definitive. A biopsy is still necessary to differentiate malignant tumor from benign.

CT SCAN OF THE NECK – this procedure is usually requested by doctors to determine the extent of spread of the tumor in the neck when his impression is that of cancer.

DEFINITIVE TREATMENT:

TOTAL THYROIDECTOMY – surgical removal of the whole thyroid usually indicated for masses of malignant cause. Complications of surgery include loss of voice.

HYPOTHYROIDISM - generalized body malaise, swelling of the ankles, face and extremities, loss of energy, retraction of the tongue, slowing of the heart (bradycardia), hypotension (lowering of blood pressure).

HYPOPARATHYROIDISM – cramps, spasms of the muscles of the, neck, and extremities, slowing of the heart. These complications are usually prevented by intake of THYROXIN tablets and PARATHYROID HORMONE.

SUBTOTAL THYROIDECTOMY – because of the different kinds of cancer, there used to be different methods of surgical procedure for different cancer. We often leave a portion of the thyroid to prevent the above complications. Due to recurrence of the cancer, we have abandoned this method and do complete removal of the thyroid.

MODIFIED RADICAL NECK DISSECTION – this is a surgical procedure done on cancer patients to remove the lymph nodes on the side of the neck in cases of cancer of the thyroid.

RADIATION OF THE NECK – radioactive therapy exposing the neck to radiation in cases of cancer of the thyroid. This is done after surgery to complete the treatment and totally eradicate the cancer cells.

MASS ABOVE THE ADAM'S APPLE

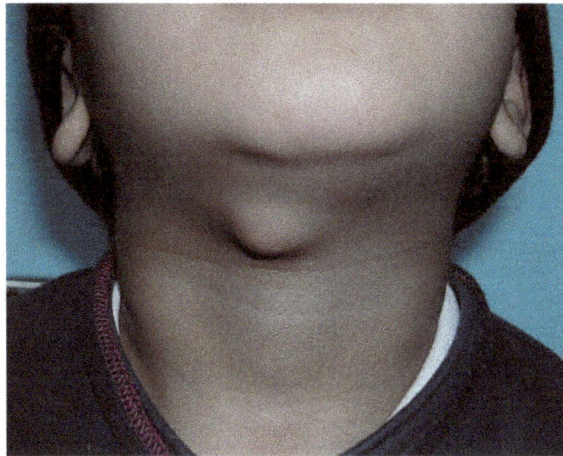

A rounded mass located above the Adam's apple in the male or female that moves on swallowing.

DIAGNOSIS: HYPOGLOSSAL DUCT CYST

ORGAN INVOLVED: *hyoid bone*

CAUSE: congenital

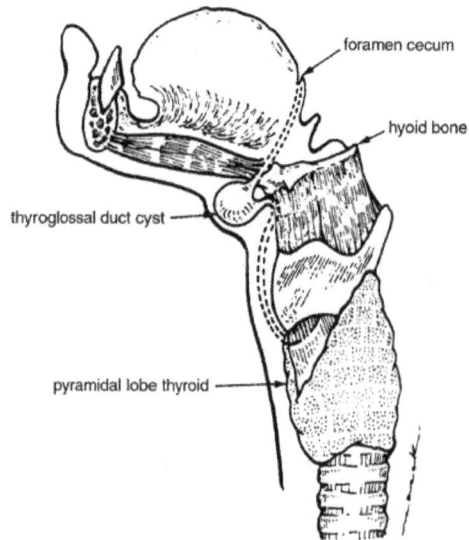

foramen cecum

hyoid bone

thyroglossal duct cyst

pyramidal lobe thyroid

INITIAL TREATMENT: none

ADVICE:

Tumors or cyst above the Adam's apple are usually present at birth but often are not noticed until the patient reaches the age of maturity. These do not give pain or disturb the patient. But at puberty, they enlarge and cause swelling.

LABORATORY EXAMINATION:

ULTRASOUND OF THE NECK – This is not necessary but often performed to determine if the tumor or cyst is an unusually located THYMUS (organ which produce the immune mechanism)

DEFINITIVE TREATMENT:

EXCISION OF THE CYST – This surgery is usually done in the operating room because the hyoid bone is cut. If the bone is left behind, the cyst recurs.

MASS UNDER THE MANDIBLE

Masses noted the mandible which are often bilateral (both sides) and are painful associated with sore throat, fever and enlarged tonsils or tooth abscess

DIAGNOSIS: ACUTE LYMPHADENITIS

ORGAN INVOLVED: *lymph nodes of the submandibular area*

CAUSE: spread of infection to the lymph nodes from the tonsils or from tooth abscess.

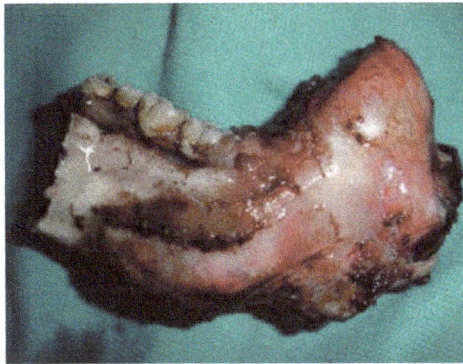

INITIAL TREATMENT:
 For adult: CLORACILLIN 500 mg 1 cap 3x a day for 7 days
 Mefenamic acid 500 mg tablet every 4 hours for pain
 For children: CLORACILLINSUSP 125 mg 1tsp 4x a day for 1 week.
 TEMPRA FORTE SUSP 1 tsp. every 4 hrs. for fever and pain

ADVICE:
 Infection in the mouth whether from tonsils, tooth, tongue or buccal mucosa (sides of the mouth) usually cause swelling of the lymph nodes located under the mandible (submandibular area). When this happens, infection is starting to spread and is prevented by the body from doing so.

LABORATORY EXAMINATION:

Culture and sensitivity of throat – this is done by swabbing a cotton bud on the surface of the throat or on the tonsils. The specimen is then brought to the laboratory and allowed to grow for 72 hours. The bacteria are then identified to facilitate the kind of antibiotic to use.

DEFINITVE TREATMENT: based on the result of the Culture and Sensitivity

MASSES AT THE SIDE OF THE NECK

Small masses palpable at the side of the neck usually found in children often with no appetite, no gain of weight

DIAGNOSIS: PRIMARY COMPLEX

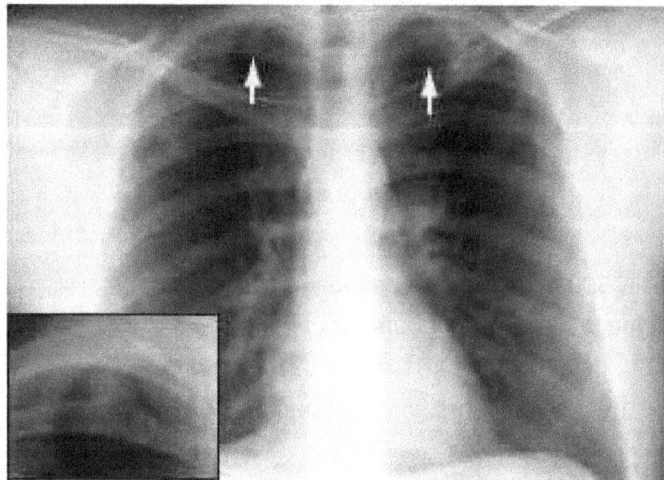

Figure 1 – Chest X-ray at two months after the onset of symptoms revealing condensation in both lung apices and mild left hilar lymph node enlargement. The insert shows the injury in the right apex.

ORGAN INVOLED: lymph nodes

CAUSE: spread of tuberculosis into the lymph nodes

INITIAL TREATMENT: none

ADVICE:

Tuberculosis of the lungs from the individuals who are living with children is the main cause of transmission. Since the bacteria can be carried airborne, any amount of closeness may cause spread of infection. Though this is not a major illness of the lungs, PRIMARY COMPLEX may be the initial symptoms of tuberculosis of the lungs. The disease is not transmitted by the use of utensils. Thus, separation of the infected individual's personal belongings is not necessary. Chest x-ray of the child may give negative results. Checkup should be done by his doctor every 3 months to determine the response of the child to the medication.

LABORATORY EXAMINATIONS:

MANTOUX TEST – this is an injection done on the skin surface of the forearm of the child. Three days after injection, the side of injection is inspected to look for any erythema or reddish discoloration surrounding the injection.

PPD Sclavo – this is another preparation of the Mantoux test which is equipped with sharp points mounted on a plastic knob. This is easier to use because it can be punctured on the forearm of a squirming child without difficulty

CHEST X-RAY – is usually negative. Sputum exam for AFB (ACID FAST BACILLI) – usually negative too.

DEFINITVE TREATMENT:

COMPRILEX SYRUP 1 tbsp. one a day for 6 months

MASS BASE OF THE NECK

Mass at the base of the neck, which is usually not accompanied by any symptom except loss of weight or slight cough.

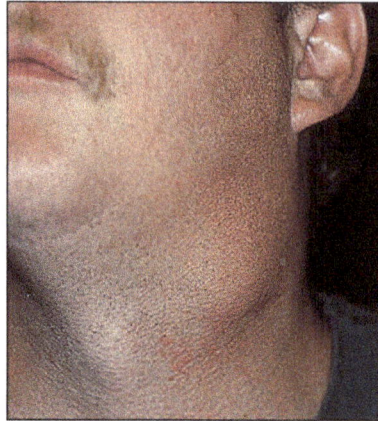

When found in women:

It may indicate infection found in the lungs or cancer in the lungs

It may indicate spread of cancer from the breast

When found in men:

It may indicate infection from the lungs, intestines, liver and other organs in the abdomen

It may indicate cancer spread from the stomach, liver and intestines

ADVICE:

When a mass or tumor is found at the base of the neck most especially on the left side, there are a lot of diseases that could cause this lymph node enlargement. The doctor's task is then to find where the primary source of infection is or the original source of cancer would be located. He will use ALL LABORATORY EXAMS in order to do so. Thus, the patient is urged to tell all the unusual symptoms he may feel or could not understand such as: episodes of sweating at night, afternoon fever, and body malaise early in the morning, frequent smoking, early satiety, loss of weight, abdominal fullness, etc., which are indicative of non-physiologic functions of the internal organs.

LABORATORY EXAMINATIONS:

PERIPHERAL SMEAR – to find any possibility of cancer of the blood (leukemia, sickle cell disease, lymphoma)

CHEST X-ray – cancer of the lungs can be seen by this examination

MAMMOGRAPHY – any changes in the substance of the breast can be detected by this exam.

ULTRASOUND OF THE LIVER – GALL BLADDER – COMMON BILE DUCT, PANCREAS AND KIDNEYS – through this examination, tumors in these areas can be detected.

DEFINITVE TREATMENT:

EXCISIONAL BIOPSY OF THE LYMPH NODE – this is the only definitive diagnostic procedure that a patient has to undergo in order to know the cause of the mass. Identification of the primary source will then give the hint as to what step should next be taken.

MASS ON THE SIDE OF THE NECK

Mass on the side of the neck which gradually enlarged the size associated with difficulty of swallowing food.

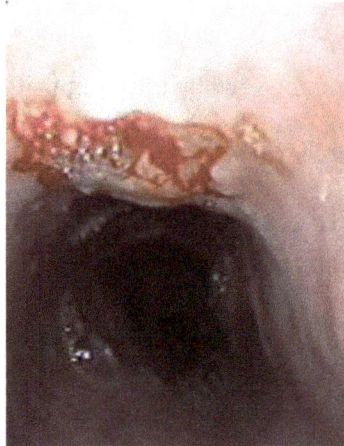

DIAGNOSIS: ESOPHAGEAL CANCER

ORGAN INVOLVED: *esophagus*

CAUSE: UNKNOWN

INITIAL TREATMENT: NONE

ADVICE:

This tumor is often found in ethnic Chinese and could not be explained why. They gradually enlarge involving the whole portion of the first part of the esophagus (food passage from the mouth to the stomach). Initially, difficulty of swallowing is the main symptom of the patient. This becomes worse until no solid food can be swallowed.

LABORATORY EXAMINATION:

BIOPSY OF THE MASS – a small piece of the tumor is excised and brought to the laboratory for examination.

CT SCAN – This is done to determine the extent of spread of the tumor.

DEFINITVE TREATMENT:

TOTAL ESOPHAGECTOMY – total removal of the upper portion of the esophagus and replace with a portion of the stomach fashioned into a tube or part of the large intestine transposed from the abdomen to the chest.

COBALT THERAPY – may extend life span.

Chapter Seven

HYPERTENSION

HYPERTENSION

At the beginning, most hypertensive does not feel anything only to discover at a routine blood pressure examination that their blood pressure is more than the normal 120/80. Starting symptoms like **headaches, dizziness**, **nuchal pains** and **palpitations** are taken for granted or interpreted as eye problem, ear problem, muscle pains and nervousness. Blood pressure readings are different for each person. One person may have 100/60 as normal and he becomes hypertensive when his blood pressure rises to 130/80. Or, he may have a blood pressure of 90/60 but he may be hypertensive if his blood pressure rises to 120/80; the normal range of almost 90% of people. Thus, blood pressure readings should not to be taken as it is when done on the first consultation. The dictum, as a rule, it is safe to undergo, at least, three blood pressure readings, is to have three blood pressure readings on different time before declaring a person as hypertensive.

CAUSES OF HYPERTENSION

1. HYPERTENSION due to kidney diseases: kidney failure, renal artery obstruction, acute glomerulonephritis to name a few.

2. HYPERTENSION secondary to high cholesterol level.

3. ESSENTIAL HYPERTENSION of which the pathophysiology is not fully understood.

Correction of the kidney problem usually brings down the blood pressure. This kind of hypertension is a minority in terms of the number of hypertensive. But this has to be ruled out when trying to find the cause of a hypertension. Thus, a person who exhibits a high blood pressure should undergo CREATININE examination to rule out the possibility of kidney problems.

HYPERTENSION secondary to high cholesterol does not often respond to anti–cholesterol drugs. This needs a partner drug to bring down the hypertension itself. More often than not, even how religious the intake of the medications is, the cholesterol does not go down significantly to warrant withdrawal of the anti-hypertensive.

The most common kind of HYPERTENSION is the ESSENTIAL HYPERTENSION. Medicine has not fully understood the pathophysiology and thus, exact causes are not pinpointed. The causes range from tension, kind of food intake, state of the arterial vessels to viscosity of the blood, pressure produced by the automatic nervous system, heart pumping factor and resistance of the blood vessels. What is important to the layman is to understand fully the importance of their medication in order to protect themselves from the complications of HYPERTENSION.

COMPLICATIONS OF HYPERTENSION

The moment a person develops hypertension, several organs of his body are affected which may lead to disability or death.

1. **STROKE** – The arteries and veins found in the brain cannot withstand any high blood pressure above normal compared to the rest of the body because they have thin and flimsy walls. Any increase of the individual's blood pressure subjects these blood vessels to rupture. In some people, a blood pressure of 180/100 could rupture any blood vessel in the brain. Rupture of these blood vessels leads to hemorrhage inside the brain, that in turn, puts pressure on the brain itself. Any amount of pressure on any part of the brain leads to paralysis or death. Whichever, the location of the blood clot is manifested by paralysis of specific part of the body.

2. **CONGESTIVE HEART FAILURE** – the heart cannot withstand prolonged pressure gradient even though it is responsible for the arterial blood pressure. The heart walls weaken and enlarge. Due to its decrease ability to pump more blood from the lungs to the rest of the body, water accumulates in the lungs, in the lower extremities and all other parts of the body.

3. **KIDNEY FAILURE** – The tubes inside the kidney are also sensitive to any increase of blood pressure. Long standing hypertension leads to destruction of the kidney followed by kidney failure.

Because of these, the importance of taking anti-hypertensive medications is emphasized here.

ANTI – HYPERTENSION AND SOME OF THE SIDE EFFECTS:

ACETAZOLAMINDE	Numbness and tingling sensation of fingers
AMLODIPINE	Headache; swelling of ankle (edema)
BENAZEPRIL	Cough and irritation of the throat
CILAZAPRIL	Coughing
DELAPRIL	Stiffness of shoulder and neck
DILTIAZEM	Insomnia
FELODIPINE	Ankle swelling
FUROSEMIDE	Increase of uric acid
GIANFAZINE	Constipation
HYDRALAZINE	Nausea and loss of appetite
HYDROCHLOROTHIAZIDE	Muscle cramps
LACIDIPINE	Frequent urination
LISINOPRIL	Diarrhea
MANIDIPINE	Shortness of breath
METHYLDOPA	Yellowish discoloration of the eyes
METOPROLOL and other BETA BLOCKERS	Decrease libido
MOXONIDINE	Dry mouth
NEFIDIPINE	Enlargement of the breast in males
NICARDIPINE	Headache
PERINDOPRIL	Cramps
PINDOLOL	Tiredness
PRAZOSIN	Incontinence
QUINAPRIL	Rhinitis and colds like reaction
RESERPINE	Nightmares
SPIRONOLACTONE	Post-menopausal bleeding
TERAZOSIN	Colds like symptoms
VALSARTAN	Coughing
VERAPAMIL	Headaches

How to manage hypertension:

1. Do not stop medication. The only time you can temporarily stop is when you know that your blood pressure is normal; that is, you have just taken your blood pressure within 6 hours.
2. Hypertensive medications have side effects. Discuss with your doctor when you have experienced these side effects. Thus, the practice of transferring from one doctor to another is hazardous.
3. Regular blood pressure determination (should be done) is once a week, if one cannot take his blood pressure every day.
4. Response to hypertensive medication varies as they are taken in a longer period of time. Shifting to another medication should be done with the advice of your physician.

Chapter Eight

Diabetes

DIABETES MELLITUS

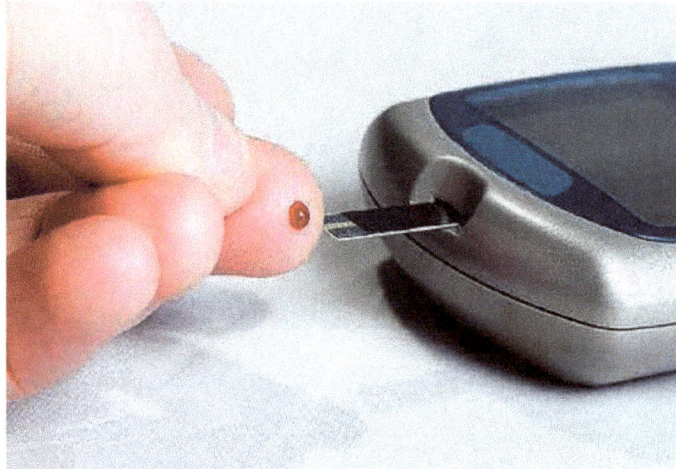

SYMPTOMS :

1. MARKED LOSS OF WEIGHT
2. FREQUENT URINATION AT NIGHT
3. DRY MOUTH AND FREQUENTLY THIRSTY
4. RECURRENT SKIN INFECTION
5. RAPIDLY EXPANDING INFECTION FROM TRUMA (i.e. punctured wound)

LABORATORY EXAMANITION:

FASTING BLOOD SUGAR – having no breakfast and no food intake starting 12 midnight.

Blood should be taken between 7 to 9 am only

- NORMAL RESULT 4.5 to 6.4

URINALYSIS – may detect spillage of sugar in the urine. It is one of the primary exams that could detect diabetes.

TREATMENT:

GLICLAZIDE 30 mg daily

METFORMIN 500 mg 3x a day

INSULIN INJECTION

COMPLICATIONS OF DIABETES:

1. DIABETIC GANGRENE – blood supply to the foot, hands and skin are blocked by diabetes.
   a. **ON SKIN** – big wound ulceration with massive darkening and death of skin.
      TREATMENT: debridement and daily dressing

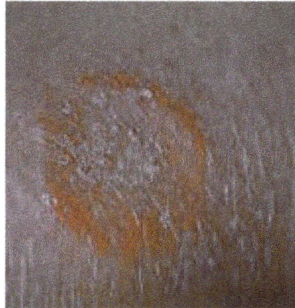

   ANTIBIOTIC: CEFUROXIME 500 mg 1 tab 3x a day until wound closes

   b. **FOOT** – darkening of the toes followed by pus formation surrounded by swelling and reddening
      TREATMENT: Amputation

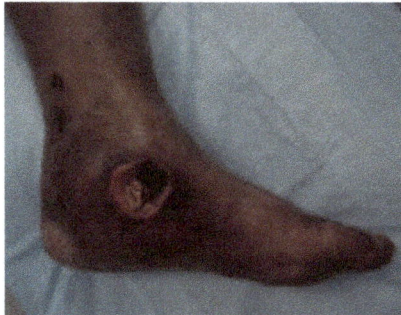

2. KIDNEY FAILURE
   a. **HEMODIALYSIS** – an ARTERIOVENOUS SHUNT is made on the arm

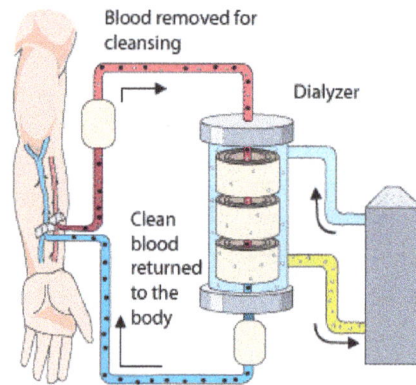

Blood removed for cleansing

Dialyzer

Clean blood returned to the body

Or like this: A – V SHUNT CATHETER to the heart

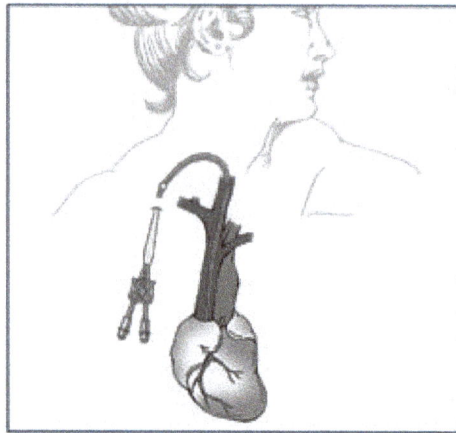

These are then connected to a HEMODIALYSIS MACHINE

b. **PERITONEAL DIALYSIS** – an incision is made below the navel and a tube is inserted through it. Fluids are then pumped inside and sucked back. Success rate is minimal unlike HEMODIALYSIS

c. **KIDNEY TRANSPLANT** – a donor must be found who is compatible with the patient. Blood examinations will be done with both donor and recipient and compatibility studies will be performed. Both donor and recipient will go to surgery at the same time with different surgical teams. Medicines will also be taken by the patient after surgery to prevent rejection of the transplanted kidney. Donor will not be harmed by the procedure except for some pains in the next 45 days after surgery. Some kidneys may be rejected but over-all, success of the transplantation is very high.

3. PERIPHERAL NEUROPATHY – diabetic patients may suffer numbness and tingling sensations on the hands and fingers. Some feel no sensation at all.

> **CAUSE**: NERVES are destroyed by diabetes.
> **INITIAL TREATMENT**: warm water immersion of affected foot 15 minutes 2x a day
> **DEFINITIVE TREATMENT**:
>> MECOBALAMINE tablet 3x a day for 3 months or more CILOSTAZOL
>> 1 tablet 3x a day for 3 months or more

4. EYE CATARACT – cataract surgery is the only treatment.
5. IMPOTENCE AND HYPOSPERMIA – some diabetic males suffer loss of libido, erectile dysfunction and low sperm count.

> **TREATMENT:**
>> SILDENAFIL CITRATE 100 mg tablet1 hr. prior to sexual intercourse
>> TESTOSTERONE UNDECANOATE 40 mg tablet 2x a day for 3 months

Chapter Nine

Smoking

SMOKING

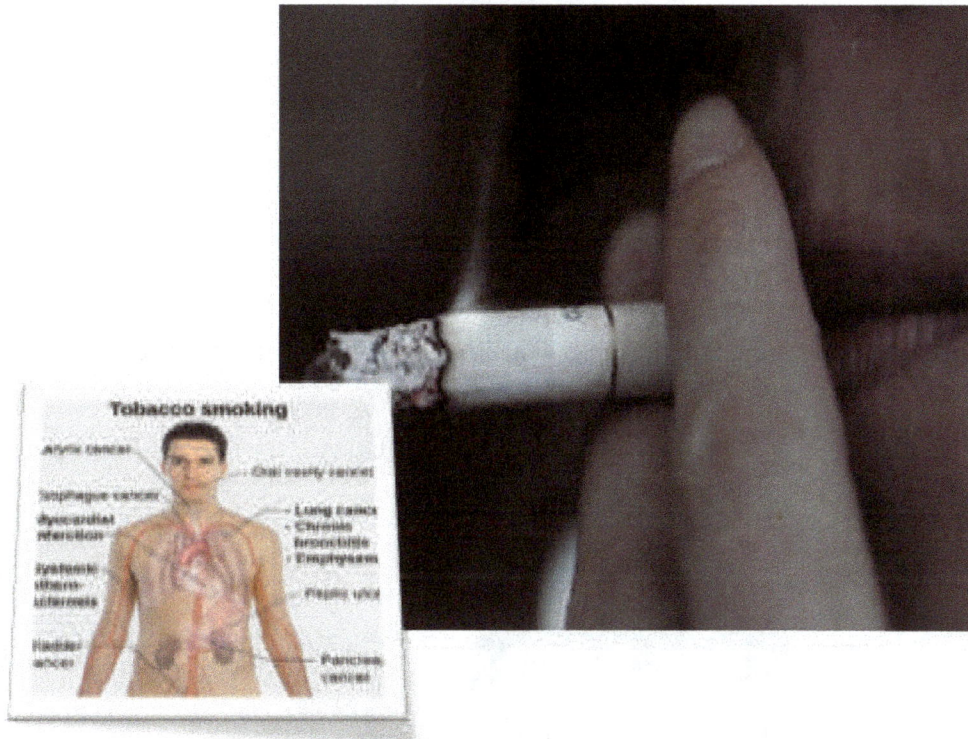

Contrary to the claims of the cigarette industry, smoking is addictive. Take it from people who have tried to stop smoking, 90% of them failed because of the urge to smoke is very strong just like illicit drugs. Many people have attempted to stop smoking earlier but they failed because their personality changes whenever, they attempted to stop smoking. Drastic change in the characteristics of the person who tries to stop smoking is very apparent, most especially, to those who have been smoking for more than ten years.

To the laymen, the destructive effect of smoking is limited to the lungs. But in my experience, smoking has done lot of destruction in so many parts of the body of the smoker.

In this chapter, pictures of destruction due to smoking will be presented, to enlighten the reader that smoking is not limited to the dysfunction of the lungs alone.

THE NORMAL LUNG

The normal lung is pinkish. Soft, fluctuant and like a sponge. It only contains air and some amount of fluid when squeezed. When squeezed, the lungs diminish in size as much 1/3 of its former size. That is how elastic it is.

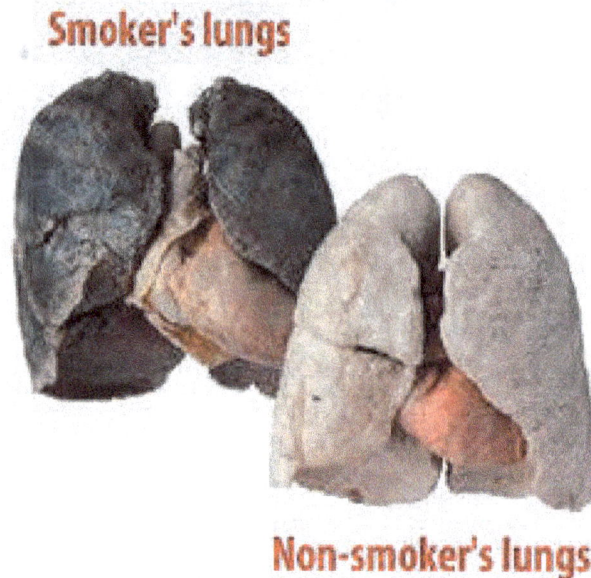

Smoker's lungs

Non-smoker's lungs

THE SMOKER'S LUNG

The smoker's lung above becomes apparent when the person has been smoking continuously for 5 years. During this time, the lung becomes black, heavy with soot, non–pliable, leathery and almost solid on its core. The owner of this lung starts to have difficulty of breathing even on slight exertion such as climbing stairs and walking briskly. He adopts a sedentary life and would prefer to sit rather than exercise which complicates the situation. Because of this, circulation of blood becomes hampered and slow to all organs of the body. This leads to further complications in the other system organs.

THE HEART IN A SMOKER

The presence of nicotine in the blood stimulates the muscles in the blood vessels (its walls are made up of smooth muscles) to constrict and narrow the lumen (diameter). This impedes the flow of blood and therefore diminishes the supply to whatever organ is involved.

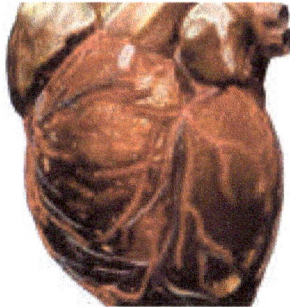

The heart is being supplied with blood vessels called coronary arteries and do not get its blood supply direct from the blood it is pumping. These coronary arteries are very sensitive to nicotine. In the presence of massive amount of nicotine, the coronary arteries constrict and close its lumen causing massive blood supply loss to the heart. This is what we call HEART ATTACK.

THE LIVER OF THE SMOKER

The main function of the liver is to detoxify whatever chemical enter the body. Nicotine is brought by blood from the lungs to the liver where it is processed. Because of its inert composition, the liver cannot detoxify nicotine and forms into black nodules scattered all over the liver parenchyma. The presence of these nodules pushes the normal cells, the veins of the liver, the arteries and the tubes that carry bile (bile ducts). These constrict and diminish the capacity of the bile ducts to drain the bile from liver to the intestine.

Thus a person who smokes ten sticks a day would have yellowish eyes, yellowish skin and yellowish areas of the body that are not exposed to the sun.

The blockade of the veins and arteries cause the liver to appear like cobblestones instead of a smooth surface. This is called HEPATIC CIRRHOSIS and limits the normal function of the liver such as production of protein and glucose necessary for the normal function of the whole body.

THE LEGS AND TOES OF A SMOKER

Like the veins and arteries in the heart and liver, these blood vessels found in the legs are affected the same way. These constrict and diminish the blood supply to the toes causing severe pain and blackening of the skin, this is called BUERGER'S DISEASE.

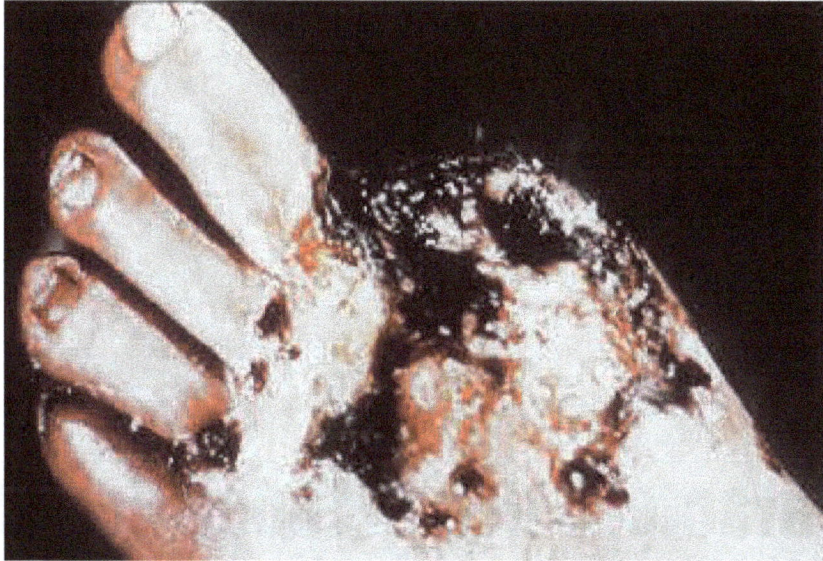

Smokers who suffer this disease prefer to cut their legs rather than stop smoking. Despite the fact, that they know the cause of their illness, and are told about it, they still continue to smoke. This confirms the addicting factor of nicotine.

All these illnesses found in the heart, lungs, liver and legs do not have any cure.

To prevent getting these illnesses - stop smoking or never start smoking!

Chapter Ten

Stool Characteristics in Loose Bowel Movement

STOOL CHARACTERISTICS IN LOOSE BOWEL MOVEMENT

FECAL CHARACTERISTICS

Observe the color, consistency, frequency and the accompanying substances found in your stools. These will indicate what disease you have.

The following chapter deals on stools and loose bowel movements. Check what color of stools, how many times you move your bowel per day, what symptoms you feel accompanying it, consistency and you will get the diagnosis by following the chart.

CONSISTENCY	COLOR	ACCOMPANYING SYMPTOM	DIAGNOSIS	TREATMENT
WATERY	YELLOW	ABDOMINAL PAIN	GASTRO ENTERITIS	SEPTRIN tablet 2x a day
WATERY	YELLOW	FEVER	ENTERO COLITIS	INOFLOX 200 2x a day
MUCOID BLOODY	BROWN	ABD PAIN BEFORE BM	AMOEBIASES	FLAGYL 500 mg 4x a day
FOOD	UNDIGESTED	ABD PAIN	INDIGESTION	HYDRASEC 1 tablet 3x a day
WATER	WHITE	DEHYDRATED	CHOLERA	KEMICETINE 500 mg 4x a day
TARRY	BLACK	PEPTIC ULCE	BLEEDING PEPTIC ULCER	PANTOLIC 40 mg daily
FORM STOOLS	GRAY	YELLOW EYES	BILIARY OBSTRUCTION	SURGERY
FORM FRESH BLOOD	BROWN	PAIN ANUS	ANAL FISSURE	FAKTU SUP 1 daily
GOAT'S STOOLS	BLACK	CONSTIPATED	COLONIC TUMOR	SURGERY
STRIPS STOOLS	BROWN	PAINFUL BOWEL	HEMORRHOIDS	DAFLON 1 tablet 3x daily
BULKY	BROWN	RAPE BOWEL MOVEMENT	HIRSCHSPRUNG	SURGERY

Chapter Eleven

Emergency Procedures

EMERGENCY PROCEDURES WHAT YOU CAN DO

In an emergency situation, the best person to help the victim is the one in front of him. It takes 5 minutes before the brain is destroyed. It takes 15 minutes or more for an emergency team to reach a victim. By this time, the victim's brain is gone and more often than not, if ever he is resuscitated, he will be in coma for a long time due to the delay.

The primary factor that is important in an emergency is for the person present in front of him not to panic. He should not run and look for help for he is the only person that could help the victim. The most logical thing to do in an emergency: PRESENCE OF MIND. Yet, it is often the most neglected thing. Presence of mind is the only thing necessary in an emergency.

The following chapter deals on all emergencies one encounters in his daily routine. Memorizing the steps would equip the reader the necessary knowledge to extend help even without any medical background.

AIR – all human beings need air. So, place the victim where he can breathe air.

BREATHING – The victim should have no obstruction to his breathing. His nose and mouth should be free from obstruction.

CIRCULATION – Circulation of blood to his brain and heart should be maintained. Any points of bleeding should be stopped.

LOSS OF CONSCIOUSNESS
IN HOT WEATHER:
1. Bringing patient away from the heat of the sun into a cold place or in the shade.
2. Let him lie down flat without pillow.
3. Place cold compress or wet towel on his armpit, inguinal area.
4. Loosen his clothes and if possible remove tight fitting clothes.
5. If consciousness is regained, let him sip small amounts of cold water.

IN FITS OF ANGER:
1. Let patient down with head prop-up with a pillow.
2. Warm compress on the chest, abdomen and thighs.
3. Take pulse to determine if present.

If Absent

> 4. Place patient without pillow.
> 5. Place open right palm on the center of the chest with open left hand on top of it.
> 6. Pump chest with jerky motion 4 times (straight elbow to be effective).
> 7. Blow air direct to the mouth of the victim.
> 8. Repeat procedure until consciousness is regained.

If Present

> 4. Do not massage or try to awaken patient. She will regain consciousness in due time.

IN HEART ATTACK:
1. Place patient flat on his back
2. Find his medicine in his pocket. If none
3. Place a tablet ISORDIL SUBLINGUAL under his tongue.
4. If none, find chili or any hot sauce in the house and rub on top his chest. Efficascent oil will do the same effect.
5. Check pulse

6. Place open palms on top of the other on the center of the chest.
7. Pump chest 4x in jerky manner (straight elbow to be effective)
8. Blow air direct into the mouth
9. Repeat procedure until pulse is detectable
10. Bring patient to hospital

If Present

6. Bring patient to hospital

IN KNOWN HYPERTENSIVE:

1. Lie patient down with head prop up with a pillow.
2. Turn head sideways to allow saliva to drip at the side of his mouth.
3. Place spoon between his teeth (tongue depressor if available)
4. Place cold compress with ice on his forehead, scalp and chest.
5. If convulsion is present, hold on to the spoon to prevent him from biting his own tongue.
6. If snoring with his saliva, turn his head almost hanging on the side of the pillow to allow all saliva to drip outside.
7. Place a tablet of CAPOTEN 25 mg under his tongue or any medications he has. If his medication is in capsule form, crush the capsule and place under his tongue.
8. Bring patient to hospital.

IN KNOWN DIABETIC:

1. Place patient flat with head lower than this chest (pillow under his back).
2. If he is semi-conscious and can understand what you are saying, ask him to chew any candy. If not, follow the next step.
3. Mix 1 tbsp. of sugar with 1 tbsp. of water and drip slowly into his mouth without choking him. Technique is to place the drip on the side of his mouth.
4. If fully conscious, bring him to the hospital.
5. If not fully conscious, repeat another tbsp. of water plus sugar.

ON A DRUNK

1. Place patient flat with head prop up with pillow.
2. Turn his head sideways to prevent aspiration of vomit.
3. Place warm compress on his head, chest, arms, and thighs.
4. Rub skin with towels soaked with warm water to redness including his chest and abdomen.
5. If consciousness is back, ask him to take a bath with warm water.

STABBED WOUNDS AND GUN SHOT WOUNDS

ON THE HEAD

1. Place thumb on the bleeding points. If larger than thumb, make a ball of cloth and place on top of the bleeding wound. Do not withdraw until he is brought to the hospital.
2. Do not place anything else on the wound (leaves, flower, whatever).

IN THE NECK

1. Place thumb DIRECTLY on top of the bleeding points but not so much to choke the patient.
2. Check if he could breathe freely with your pressure.
3. Check if blood is present in his mouth:

If Blood is Present

4. More pressure on the bleeding point.
5. Turn his head sideways to drip blood on the side of his mouth.
6. Bring patient to hospital.

> 4. Light thumb pressure or just adequate enough to stop bleeding.
> 5. Bring patient to hospital.

ON THE CHEST BUT NOT MUCH BLEEDING

1. Plug stabbed wound entry with anything (ball of cloth, handkerchief, gloves, and rubber). Plugging is adequate when the sucking noise produced when the patient inhales stops.
2. Place patient flat with head lower than the chest or the rest of the body.
3. Bring patient to the hospital.

ON THE CHEST WITH SPURTING BLOOD

1. Pack wound with a ball of cloth and pressure with hand.
2. If available, tie legs and arms with rubber bonds or rope to redirect blood back to the heart.
3. Rush to the nearest hospital.

ON THE ABDOMEN

1. Place back intestines inside abdomen if possible and pack wound with cloth.
2. Rush to the hospital.

ON THE THIGHS AND ARMS

1. Place ball of cloth directly on the top of the bleeding point.
2. Do not place tourniquet above or below the wound.
3. Tie the ball of cloth just enough to stop the bleeding and not so tight to restrict blood flow to the arms or legs.
4. Check pulse on the wrist or near the ankle to determine blood flow before transfer to hospital.

DROWNING

1. Place patient on a hard flat surface with head lower than the rest of the body.
2. Place both open hands on the center of the chest.

3. Push 4x with a jerky motion (elbow should be straight to be effective).
4. Close nostrils patient coughs out water AND IS FULLY CONSCIOUS. Do not stop when patient half regains consciousness or moans. DO NOT TRANSFER OR TRANSPORT TO HOSPITAL UNTIL PATIENT IS FULLY CONSCIOUS. Most victims die on the way to the hospital when resuscitation is inadequately done. Anyone can do this. The person who is most aggressive to do it must continue and should not be replaced.

CONVULSION

1. Place patient flat with head turn sideways.
2. Insert spoon (tongue depressor if available) in between the teeth forcefully.
3. CHECK TEMPERATURE.

If with Fever

4. Pack armpits, inguinal, neck, chest, with ice.
5. Sponge patient with water soaked towels until skin becomes reddish.
6. Chip ice into small bits and insert into anus (if child). Careful not to insert sharp ones.
7. Repeat above until patient stops convulsing.

If NO Fever

4. Hold on to arms and legs to prevent fractures.
5. Consult a neurologist.

BURNS

OPEN FLAME AND SCALDING

1. Immerse affected part of the body in cold water until the pain subsides. Cold compress may help if there is no large amount of water.
2. Do not remove bullae or parts of skin that forms into globes.

3. Place FLAMMAZINE CREAM into clean gauze bandage in thin layers.
4. Apply the impregnated gauze on the affected area and press.
5. Place another layer of clean gauze bandage without FLAMMAZINE on top of the first layer.
6. Hold the bandage by applying a ROLLER GAUZE BANDAGE if the affected area is the arm or legs. If it is on the body, plasters will hold it.
7. Change of dressings should be done daily. Pouring HYDROGEN PEROXIDE on the bandage will help in removing the soiled bandages. Ordinary water could do the same trick.
8. DO NOT APPLY FLAMMAZINE CREAM direct to the burned area. This form into a thick scab preventing faster healing and promotes infection.
9. ANTIBIOTICS: CLOXACILLIN 500 mg 1 cap 3x a day for 10 days.
10. ANALGESICS: MEFENAMIC ACID 500 mg 1 cap every 4 hours.
11. Apply dressings daily until wounds are dry (5 – 7 days).
12. To diminish scarring. Apply CONTRACTUBEX cream for 3 months.

ELECTRICAL BURNS
1. Pour cold water direct to the wound for 15 minutes.
2. Wash with soap and water to remove burned tissues and skin.
3. Dry wound with clean cloth or bandage.
4. Place FLAMMAZINE CREAM on a piece of bandage and cover wound with it.
5. Place gauze without FLAMMAZINE on top of the first layer.
6. Fix with plaster or roller gauze bandage.
7. Daily dressing for 5 – 7 days.

CHOKING

FOR ADULT
1. Stand at the back of the patient.
2. Embrace patient at the level of his navel (umbilicus).
3. Press his abdomen with a jerky motion. Raising him suddenly by his belly will also do the trick.

FOR CHILDREN
1. Place child on your lap face downwards with head lower than his buttocks.
2. Press abdomen with a jerky motion. Repeat until chocking material is coughed out.

Chapter Twelve

Wound Care

AFTER MINOR OPERATION

Pain sets in after every operation. The anesthesia will only last for 1 hour and a half. So, you need to take analgesics (paracetamol, mefenamic acid, diclofenac) every four hours. Even if it is not aching, you have to take the medicine because it will take another thirty minutes for it to take effect. If you don't want pain, take it; take it even if you are not prodded by a celebrity endorser.

Take a bath. You don't want doctors to smell your most innermost secrets, do you? It has nothing to do with your wound. We even wash your intestine when we do major surgeries in your tummy, how much more a small wound in your breast, on your arm, on your face or on your anus? The more you wash it, the fewer bacteria you need to kill with antibiotics. You have to take off the bandage, of course. If you don't want it toasting, keep it covered while taking a bath. After you wash, take it off and replace with a dry bandage. Band-Aid will do. There is no need for betadine. If you can tolerate the pain, wash your wound with soap and water, it is the best.

You can eat anything. You would just add to the economic boom hoax. What you eat will not go to the wound as is. If you eat wild pig, it would not be the wild pig that would go to your wound. An eggplant does not do harm to your wound, either, unless, of course, you use it for rubbing your back. Dried salted fish does not cause itchiness to the wound. It is the wound that is itching and not the dried salted fish. After 5 days it will heal even if you don't go to a healing crusade.

The bandage is not part of your make up. It does not have to be changed every day nor does it have to be rearranged like your skirt or your panty. The purpose of the bandage is to catch the sipping blood from the wound, which is more likely, when your operation is bloody. When the bandage becomes wet, that is the time you have to change your bandage.

Most of the minor operations I do, I always close it with absorbable sutures, which means, we do not have to remove the sutures. It dissolves. Hence, you need not return to have an update about it. The only time you have to return is when you bring with you the result of the biopsy (usually ten days). Both you and I are interested to see whether you are going to live for the next ten years.

Rain showers and thunderstorms have something to do with your wound. If it is cold, your wound aches even if it is healed or has been there for the last two years. Why? Like all the muscles of your body, cold weather causes contraction in your wound. Hence, the surrounding tissues of your wound are non-tensile anymore. This means, that during muscle contraction, the whole scar moves causing pressure on the nerves which results to pain. You need no tablets, lotions or any powder to ease the pain. A simple caress on the wounded part will give relief.

If your doctor asks you to come back to the clinic, please do so. It has something to do with your wound. Either, he has to remove the drain that he placed there or remove the sutures he used during major operation because they are not absorbable. In my case, I have to use the non-absorbable suture because there is tension in your wound and would not close properly with an absorbable one.

INDEX OF DIAGNOSIS

ALKALINE PHOSPHATASE – blood exam that determines any disease found only in the common bile duct and infection is one of them.

ALPHAFETO PROTEIN – examination of the blood, which confirms the presence of cancerous tumors in the liver based on the high level of immune protein enzymes.

ASO TITER – blood examination to determine whether the sore throat infection may lead to RHEUMATIC HEART DISEASE.

BARIUM ENEMA – administration of a milk-like substance into the anus prior to taking x-rays of the abdomen. Several films are taken in different angles to locate the tumor.

BIOPSY OF THE HEMORRHOIDAL MASS – it is necessary to screen out the possibility of malignancy presented by any anal mass such as hemorrhoids.

BLOOD PRESSURE DETERMINATION - to rule out HYPERTENSION most especially in the older age group.

BLOOD URIC ACID DETERMINATION – to determine the level of uric acid, which is the common cause of gouty arthritis.

BREAST SONOGRAM – may be of use to determine the presence of masses that contain liquid and less likely to produce a radiation exposure. False negative is greater. False positive is more likely. It is valuable in differentiating solid tumors from cystic tumors.

BRONCHIAL WASHINGS – through bronchoscopy (a fiber-optic tube used to visualize the inside of the bronchus) pieces of the bronchus are taken for the laboratory examination. The tube is inserted direct to the bronchus with the patient half-awake or generally anesthetized. Diagnostics accuracy is minimal if the lesion is in the lungs and not in the tubes (bronchus).

BRONCHOSCOPY – patient is sedated or generally anesthetized. A tube is inserted through the nose into the stomach to prevent regurgitation of food into the lungs. A fiber-optic tube is directly inserted into the bronchus and a long forceps grasps the coin.

CHEST X-RAY – is a definitive laboratory exam that could determine presence of phlegm in the lungs. But in some cases, due to the small amount of the phlegm in the lungs, only with the use of the stethoscope by a physician could determine this lung problem.

Fluid is shown on x-ray as whitening otherwise black area in an aerated lung. When small in amount, it usually pools in the side of the lungs near the diaphragm and is describe as BLUNTING OF THE COSTOPHERICAL ANGLE. When the amount of fluid is great, a wide part of the lateral side of the lungs is covered by a whitish on x-ray film.

COLONOSCOPY – a flexible hose-like instrument the size of the small finger with light source of its own. The fiber-optic tube is about 5 feet in length and can reach the uppermost portion of the large intestine. Visualization is done directly and thru TV monitor. Biopsy can be performed with the instrument gadgetry.

COLONOSCOPY – FIBER-OPTIC – this is done using a thin tube the size of the small finger, inserted into the anus and guided manually up to the whole length of the large intestine. Visualization is done through a TV monitor and/or through the fiber-optic tube.

COMPLETE BLOOD COUNT (CBC) – to determine the presence of infection anywhere in the body though not specific for acute appendicitis. Any increase of the white blood cells above 10,000 and in the absence of any other focus of infection such as in the Upper Respiratory tract is indicative of Acute Appendicitis.

CORONARY ANGIOGRAM – use to determine the location and extent of the blocked blood vessels of the heart. A small tube is inserted through a vein in the arm or neck and threaded direct into the heart. A dye is injected and an x-ray is done at the same time.

CREATININE – blood exam to determine the current status of kidney function. This is very important in determining the extent of damage done by stone or infection. Patient must not eat beginning midnight until the blood is extracted before 9 am the next day.

CREATININE CLEARANCE – blood examination to determine status of the kidney before surgery.

CREATININE CLEARANCE DETERMINATION – blood examination to determine function of the kidney.

CT SCAN – a diagnostic work up to determine the respectability of the lesion (whether patient can benefit by radical surgery). Biopsy of the lesion may be done with the guide of this modality.

CT SCAN OF THE NECK – is the best diagnostic tool to look for blood vessel injuries.

CT SCAN OF THE ABDOMINALCAVITY – hemorrhage and pooling of blood in the abdomen can be detected by this procedure. Any injury to the liver and spleen no matter how small it is can be seen by this exam.

CT SCAN OF THE BRAIN – use to determine the location of the blood clot and possible surgical removal.

CT SCAN OF THE CRANIUM – diagnosis could only be attained through the use of this diagnostic tool. Location and the size of the tumor are definitely attained and the procedure is not invasive and traumatic to the patient. Planning for surgery could also be accomplished and the possibility of complete surgical removal could also be evaluated.

CT SCAN OF THE THORAX – small lesions of the lungs in their early stage could be detected. But routine examination with the use of this diagnostic stool is very expensive.

CULTURE AND SENSITIVITY – a laboratory exam use to isolate the bacteria and determine the antibiotic most effective against it. This is most frequently necessary when the infection is resistant to common treatment and symptoms persist despite adequate antibiotics.

CYTOLOGY EXAM OF SPUTUM – some lung cancers can be diagnosed through this method. This is done by collecting all the sputum expectorated by the patient in 24 hours. Lung cancer detection is not accurate. Many are missed by this method.

DENGUE RAPID TEST – recently launched exam for dengue but is not 100% accurate. Some may give false negative results or false positive results.

ECG – ELECTROCARDIOGRAM – is the fastest way of diagnosing heart attacks. Electrical wirings are attached to the chest connected to a machine, which reads the electrical impulse generated by the heart. Abnormalities of the lines created by the machine indicate diseases like a heart attack.

ENDOCOSPIC PROSTATIC BIOPSY – through a tube with light source, the prostate is visualized via the penile shaft and a piece of tissue is removed and examine in the laboratory.

ESOPHAGOGRAM – x-ray procedure whereby the patient is asked to swallow milky substance and x-ray is taken in the act of swallowing. This may visualize stricture or mass inside the esophagus. Not diagnostic in terms of determining malignancy.

ESOPHAGOSCOPY – both diagnostics as well as therapeutic. In some cases, due to massive bleeding, the procedure may not stop bleeding due to visual difficulty.

FASTING BLOOD SUGAR – determines the presence of diabetes.

FINE NEEDLE BIOPSY – a long needle is inserted into the right upper quadrant of the abdomen (RUQ) direct to the liver and a sample is aspirated and brought to the laboratory. This is the definitive diagnostic exam to classify which tumor is malignant or benign.

GASTROSCOPY + BIOPSY – a long fiber-optic is inserted through the mouth into the stomach visualizing the tumor or ulcer. Biopsy of the suspected area is done to confirm the diagnosis.

GASTROSCOPY – a special procedure wherein a very thin tube with a light on the tip (fiber-optic) is inserted into the mouth down to the stomach to visualize the ulcer. The patient must not eat anything in the morning until the exam is done. The result can be seen on TV monitor and a direct biopsy (a piece of the stomach is taken) can be done subsequently. The procedure may trigger wreathing.

GRAM STAINS OF STOOLS - to determine the specific bacterium causing the loose bowel movement.

GRAM STRAINING OF THROAT – throat swab done on the pharynx to isolate the bacteria responsible.

H. PYLORI DETERMINATION – blood exam to determine if H. pylori (kind of bacteria responsible for causing peptic ulcer) are present.

HEMOGLOBIN AND HEMATOCRIT – is a blood concentration tests necessary to monitor.

HEPATITIS B SURFACE ANTIGEN – determines exposure to Hepatitis B infection or vaccination. Most foreign countries require overseas foreign workers to be negative to this test. Person's positive to this test will not be employed.

INTRAVENOUS PYELOGRAM – the most accurate x-ray examination to pinpoint the location of the stone in the ureter.

- An x-ray procedure done by injecting a chemical (contrast media) into the vein in the arm. Several x-ray views and positions are taken in different minute interval. This will show the size of the kidney, it's inside structure, stones inside the kidney if present, the ureter (tube connecting the kidney to the urinary bladder) and the urinary bladder.

LARYNGEAL BIOPSY OF THE TUMOR – this requires bronchoscopy where a tube is inserted directly to the throat and the mass remove by a long instrument. This is then brought to the laboratory for microscopic examination. Anesthesia is local spray and does not usually require general anesthesia for some patients.

LIPID PROFILE – determines cholesterol which may be one of the causes of hypertension.

LUMBAR TAP – aspiration of the brain fluid (CEREBRO-SPINAL FLUID) done at the back of the patient at the level of the lumbar vertebrae. Though the procedure is innocuous, accidental brain herniation may occur when there is a concomitant high cranial pressure. The fluid is brought to the laboratory to determine the presence of bacterial infection.

MAGNETIC RESONANCE IMAGING (MRI) – the complete examination of the spinal cord injury. It uses polarizing magnets to visualize any part of the body. Radiation is minimal compared to x-rays. 3D examination results are possible completely visualizing the extent of injury. With this modality, surgical planning can be completely done prior to intervention.

MAMMOGRAPHY – done in women whose family history is positive for CANCER (mother, aunt, grandparents).

- Has to be done if no masses are palpable in the breast to screen out the possibility of non-palpable tumors (less than 5mm).

MRI – is the most definitive diagnostic tool to determine other possible damage to the bone joint. Otherwise it has negative findings.

PAPS SMEAR – routine diagnostic exam to determine any cancer of the cervix and uterus. This is done by scraping the surface of the cervix with a wooden spatula.

PERIPHERAL SMEAR – to determine blood dyscrasias and other blood related diseases like leukemia, anemia.

PERITONEAL LAVAGE – A small incision is made below the navel under local anesthesia. A tube is inserted through the wound and several liters of dextrose water are poured into the abdomen through this tube. After several minutes, the water is suctioned back and examined for traces of blood and feces the presence of which indicate injury of the intestines and abdominal organs.

PLATELET COUNT – Normal is above 150,000. Any rapid decrease in the count indicates DENGUE FEVER.

PROCTOSIGMOIDOSCOPY – a rigid instrument the size of a thumb and 20cm long is inserted into the anus. Visualization of the inside of the anus is done directly with the patient lying on his side. Discomfort is felt when the scope reaches the uppermost portion of the large intestine. Biopsy of any lesion found on examination can be done using long limbed pliers-like instrument called alligator forceps. No pain is felt but minimal bleeding may occur and blood can be noticed in stools for 24 hours.

PROCTOSIGMOIDOSCOPY – RIGIDSCOPE – this is a half inch tube with a light source about 20 inches in length and inserted direct to the anus to visualize inner portion of the anus and the distal portion of the large intestines. It has a limited range and therefore not ideal to examine the whole of the large intestine.

PROSTATIC SERUM ASSAY – determines the presence of prostate cancer.

RECTAL EXAMINATION – it is an examination of the anus with index finger with a minimal amount of discomfort. Most lesions are found thru this simple examination.

SGPT / SGOT – blood examinations to determine liver functions

SPUTUM EXAM FOR ACID FAST BACILLI – collection of sputum in 24-hour period and submission of the specimen in the laboratory. This will identify the bacterium responsible for Tuberculosis.

STOOL EXAM – to determine the possibility of other cross infections like amoeba, parasitism, etc.

TYPHIDOT – blood exam which is more accurate and fast than WIDAL TEST but more expensive.

ULTRASOUND – sound is directed to the kidney-ureter-urinary bladder. The backfire of this sound will be reflected in a TV-like monitor giving the silhouette of these structures, which determine the extent of infection, kidney damage and to rule out the possibility of kidney stones.

ULTRASOUND (2D ECHOCARDIOGRAM) – only used to determine valvular and anatomic cardiac defects.

ULTRASOUND OF THE GALL BLADDER – it is a definitive diagnostic exam that could differentiate the disease from any other forms of abdominal pain. This is done in consonance with ultrasound of the liver, common bile duct, pancreas and kidneys to determine possible disease entities in these areas, which may present the same symptoms. Patient should not take any food from midnight until the procedure is done at 8 am.

ULTRASOUND OF THE KIDNEY- URETER-URINARY BLADDER – the fastest, cheapest and safest way to diagnose kidney stones.

ULTRASOUND OF THE LIVER – tumors of the liver of any kind can detect by this method. But it does not classify which is cancerous and which is benign.

ULTRASOUND OF THE LIVER AND SPLEEN – the fastest way to diagnose any injury to the liver or spleen.

ULTRASOUND OF THE LIVER, GALL BLADDER, COMMON BILE DUCT AND PANCREAS – yellowish discoloration of the eyes and skin has so many causes. It is only through this examination that defines diagnosis that could be accomplished in short time.

ULTRASOUND OF THE PROSTATE – will indicate enlargement of the prostate.

ULTRASOUND OF THE SCROTUM – this is done to rule out the possibility of other illnesses, which may manifest as pain in the scrotum. Otherwise, no definitive finding is found in cases like this.

ULTRASOUND OF THE UTERUS AND ADNEXEA – the cheapest way to diagnose any tumor in the uterus. This can be done transvaginal (probe is inserted into the vagina) or transabdominal (above the abdomen).

UPPER GI SERIES – a special kind of x-ray wherein the patient is asked to drink a milk –like substance after which an x-ray of the abdomen is done. The patient is asked not to eat anything starting midnight up to the time of x-ray. X-ray films are taken in different positions (patient is asked to lie flat, prone, and sideways) in a dark room. All street clothes will be taken off and a hospital gown is used during the procedure.

UPRIGHT FILM OF THE ABDOMEN – An x-ray is taken with the patient standing up or the x-ray table is tilted upwards. This is done to bring down water in the intestine to level off. Presence of water leveling off inside the intestine similar to the steps of a ladder signifies intestinal obstruction.

URETHRAL SMEAR – with the use of a glass slide, a smear of the penile discharge is examined. The bacteria are identified using this method.

URIC ACID DET – examination of the blood after fasting post-midnight

URINALYSIS – cheapest way to determine infection in the urinary tract.

WIDAL TEST – blood examination, which detects presence of Typhoid in the blood.

X-RAY – use to be the diagnostic tool before the advent of ultrasound. Medicines (contrast media) are given a day prior to the exam to visualize the gall bladder.

X-RAY OF THE ABDOMEN – can only indicate that intestines are side-swept or set aside by pus or in ileus (intestines are not moving) because of infection. Some may show fecalith or stony feces near the base of the appendix. It does not help in the diagnosis.

X-RAY OF THE CERVICAL VERTEBREA / LUMBO-SACRAL VERTEBREA – x-rays done on the neck or back to determine the extent of injury. It only shows the fractures where the involved vertebra is located. It does not show the extent of injury to the spinal cord.

X-RAY OF THE LUMBAR VERTEBRA – to determine the extent of stiffening of the lumbar bones and the presence of any spondylitic spike formation.

- to determine if the bone joint is grossly affected

X-RAY OF THE NECK – presence of air in the subcutaneous tissue indicates penetration but does not pinpoint the injured structure.

X-RAY OF THE THORACIC BONY CAGE – to determine the magnitude of swelling or the presence of it; fractures could also be detected.

X-RAY OF THE THORACIC VERTEBRA – to determine the extent of the bone destruction and necessity of surgery for debridement and reconstruction.

INDEX OF SURGICAL PROCEDURES

APPENDECTOMY - An operation done on the right lower quadrant of the abdomen. A small incision is made at the right side below the umbilicus, which could be horizontal or oblique depending on the surgeon who is doing it. With the appendix right down below the incision, it is pulled up. The base of the appendix is cut and ligated (tied) with an absorbable suture. All pus pooling near the appendix is sucked out and bleeders are also tied. The abdomen is closed layer by layer (4 layers: peritoneum, muscles, fatty layer and skin). Based on what is found inside, the location where the intestine is knotting is cut and sutured back together.

BETAMETHASONE INTRATHECAL INJECTION or on the site of pain – immediate relief of pain is usually accomplished.

   - Bloated abdomen

BRONCHOSCOPY – patient is sedated or generally anesthetized. A tube is inserted through the nose into the stomach to prevent regurgitation of food into the lungs. A fiber-optic tube is directly inserted into the bronchus.

- Visualization of bleeding points needs an experienced Pulmonologist. In good hands, procedure is easy and fast. Cauterization of the bleeding points is the only procedure that can be done to stop bleeding.

CHEST TUBE INSERTION – surgical opening of a wound in the space between ribs and insertion of a large tube to drain the fluid into water-sealed bottle- a simple bottle containing water, which prevents air from entering while catching the drainage from the chest.

CHEST TUBE INSERTION (THORACOSTOMY) – the opening on the side of the chest and insertion of a tube into the chest cavity for drainage of HEMOTHORAX AND PNEUMOTHORAX. The chest tube is attached to a bottle filled with 2 inches of water where the other end of the tube is immersed to prevent air to escape from entering into the lungs during inspiration but allow air to escape from the lungs in expiration.

CHOLECYTOSTOMY – It is the relief of the bile obstruction by opening the gall bladder and draining it out thru a skin opening. This is a temporary procedure just to relieve the obstruction. A definitive surgery will follow when the patient faces the crisis.

CHOLEDOCO-DUODENOSTOMY – It is the short-circuiting of the common bile duct by attaching it direct to the duodenum – a portion of the small intestine next to stomach.

CHOLEDOCO- JEJUNOSTOMY – it is short-circuiting of the common bile duct by attaching it direct to the jejunum – a part of the small intestine distal to the stomach.

CHOLEDOCOSTOMY – The process of creating an opening into the common bile duct for drainage.

COBALT TREATMENT – is a radiation therapy used for cancer treatments. It destroys tumors spreading near the voice box and adds more years.

COLONIC RESECTION – it is the removal of a segment of the large intestine with preservation of the community of the intestine (end to end anastomosis).

COMPLETE JOINT REPLACEMENT – involving the replacement of the normal bone joint with composite made materials like titanium, ceramics, plastic resins, and stainless steel. This is a major surgery, crutches for months and instability for weeks.

CONSTRICTION OF THE ANAL CANAL – the hole of the anus may become small causing discomfort or pain on defecation. This may require dilatation under spinal anesthesia if bowel movement is greatly affected.

CORONARY BYPASS – it is a surgical procedure wherein a vein from the thigh of the patient is transplanted into the heart to bypass a clogged portion similar to a "flyover" road complex.

CORONARY STENT – a spring-like small contraption is inserted through a vein in the neck and threaded into the coronaries of the heart to open up the clogged portion of the artery. No major surgical procedure is done but a small wound is made in the neck where the instrument is inserted to carry the "spring" to the heart.

CRANIOTOMY – complete removal of tumor is the objective of surgery. Malignancy limits the prognosis and of possible cure and is therefore of extreme importance to be taken into consideration when contemplating surgery. After surgery, the paralysis may persist and could not be alleviated. Therefore, this should be thoroughly discussed between the relatives and the surgeon in order to understand the outcome of the procedure.

DEBRIDEMENT – removal of the pus formations by sharp dissection after application of local anesthesia such as MLAC.

DEBRIDEMENT AND SUTURING – if the wound is more than sharp 2 cm, suturing should be done to approximate the edges. They heal faster and complications are lesser.

DIAMOND TECHNIQUE - piecemeal removal of the hemorrhoids with diamond shape incisions made longitudinal to the anal canal. No severe complications but recurrence is very high.

DRAINAGE OF THE SINUSES - this is accomplished by actual pumping of the sinus chambers thru the nose. The procedure is very uncomfortable and patient may feel like drowning.

DRESSING – application of wound ointments embedded dressings such as SILVER SULFADIAZINE.

ESOPHAGECTOMY – total removal of the esophagus from the base of the mouth to the stomach through an incision on the side of the chest. Continuity of the intestine is made by using a segment of the large intestine as esophagus or a portion of the stomach fashioned into a tube and attached to the remaining portion of the throat.

ESOPHAGOSCOPY (GASTROSCOPY) – a fiber-optic tube is inserted into the mouth to examine the whole length of the esophagus. Fulguration (burning) of bleeding points can be done with this instrument. Before the advent of this instrument, exploration of the esophagus was usually done by surgery with a wound made on the chest extending from the back to the front. This was indicated in patients who develop massive bleeding from the esophagus.

EXCISIONAL BIOPSY – it is the removal of entire breast mass under local anesthesia and sending of the specimen to the laboratory. The result takes 7 to 10 days to be available. Definitive removal of entire mass is done. False negative absolutely none.

EXPLORATION OF THE ESOPHAGUS – this is done by making an opening on the abdomen by surgery, going through the stomach and suturing the bleeding points in the gastro-esophageal junction.

EXPLORATION OF THE NECK WOUND – under general anesthesia, the wound is widened and the big blood vessels of the neck are examined for possible injury. Immediate closure of these wounds is done with the use of vascular sutures. Injuries to the bronchial structures may not need further treatment unless they are causing difficulty of breathing to the patient. When it is causing difficulty breathing, a temporary TRACHEOSTOMY is done. TRACHEOSTOMY is an emergency procedure wherein a wound is made below the Adam's apple and the windpipe (bronchus) is exposed. An opening is made on the bronchus itself and a tracheostomy tube (a curve metal tube) is inserted to serve as an airway inlet-outlet. This procedure is difficult to do without proper instruments and lighting and should never be attempted outside of the hospital setting.

EXPLORATORY LAPAROTOMY – it is a general term to describe surgical opening of the abdomen to determine the cause of an illness.

An operation done for acute appendicitis which have ruptured or the diagnosis is vague but the symptoms of the patient warrant surgery. Acute Abdomen – term describing an abdominal situation which medical treatment cannot correct and only an operation can save the patient). The incision is made from the top of the abdomen (epigastric) down to the lower portion of the abdomen (hypogastric). All parts of the abdomen is inspected and cleaned (in ruptured Appendicitis) by pouring water inside the abdomen. Appendectomy proper (as described above) is done.

EXTRACORPOREAL SOUND WAVE LITHOTRIPSY – a blast of sound is directed towards the urinary bladder to break the stone. This is often done in several courses most especially in big stones.

FINE NEEDLE BIOPSY – a large bore needle is used to extract a piece of the breast mass and send to the laboratory for diagnosis. This can be done in clinic setting; expense is very minimal. But the result usually can be available in 7 to 10 days. A second procedure has to be done in order to remove the mass if it is found to be benign. But this technique is more advantageous in that the patient can be psychologically prepared before the definitive treatment of removing the entire breast. False negative is high due to inability to sample all areas of the breast mass.

FISTULA IN ANU – formation of canals in areas of surgery.

FISTULECTOMY – it is the removal of the entire length of the canal. Visualization of the canal is highlighted with the use of methylene blue solution. Excision of the entire canal is subsequently done. Recurrence is high if the fistulous tract is not completely removed.

FROZEN SECTION – the breast mass is removed under general anesthesia and immediately sent to the laboratory to determine the presence of malignancy with the intention of doing definitive treatment of breast malignancy in one set-up (removal of the entire breast). The advantage of this set-up is that diagnosis is immediately known; anxiety is minimized; and it is cheaper. The disadvantage with this technique is that the patient is asleep and cannot be informed of the procedure.

GASTRECTOMY - removal of the stomach (partial or total) with the intention of removing the whole tumor and its surrounding tissues. Continuity of the **GASTROINTESTINAL TRACT** - is done through creation of a new stomach coming from a portion of the small intestines.

HEMICOLECTOMY – it is the removal of the involved portion of the large intestines leaving the anus intact for possible reattachment in the near future. Patient has to pass through a colostomy stage wherein the proximal end of the large intestine is brought out through an incision on the left side of the abdomen and where the patient moves his feces temporarily via a colostomy bag.

HEPATIC LOBECTOMY – a lobe of the liver is totally removed. This is only indicated if the cancer is confined to one lobe. Presence of metastasis (spread) does not warrant this operation.

HERNIORRHAPHY – repair of the abdominal wall defect by closure of the inguinal canal. 4 -7 days hospital stay. Healing period 45 days to 2 months.

HUMAN ANTI-TETANUS IMMUNE GLOBULIN 250 u im– for immediate coverage against tetanus if patient has never been given tetanus vaccination in the past or for the last ten years. This injection only last for 30 days.

HYSTERECTOMY – removal of the uterus, which can be done either through the vagina to give a cosmetic effect (VAGINAL HYSTERECTOMY).

INCISION AND DRAINAGE – draining with a small lancet after local anesthesia. A small rubber drain is inserted to prevent premature closure of the wound. Dressing is necessary the next day to remove the rubber drain.

INCISION AND DRAINAGE OF THE LATERAL CHAMBERS - making an incision inside the mouth through the upper molars and drainage of the sinuses.

LAMINECTOMY – surgical removal of the impinging bone in the involved lumbar vertebra thereby realizing the nerve affected. Instability of the vertebral column may result. Long physiotherapy is necessary.

LAPAROSCOPIC CHOLECYSTECTOMY – 3 small incisions are made: above the umbilicus, below it and at the side. Operation is done with the use of a laparoscope – a small tube used to visualize the gall bladder inside the abdomen without incising a big wound. Less postoperative pain means fast recovery. Technique cannot be used if the gall bladder is infected, bloated or in the presence of severe peritonitis (infection of the whole abdomen). Some procedures may be reverted to the open method due to difficulty of the procedure. Thus, expense may be added. 3 to 5 days hospital stay is a must. Recovery period would last from 10 to 15 days.

LITHOPREXY – nonsurgical and involves bombardment of kidney stones by ultrasonic device. COST: P120, 000 TO P130, 000. Repeat procedures may have to be done to dissolve stones. Failure cases are common. Side effects such as liver laceration and organ hematoma occur.

LOBECTOMY – surgical removal of a portion of the liver affected by the cancer if it still localized. If it is affecting the whole liver, liver transplantations are being experimented. Survival rate is 3 to 6 months.

LOBECTOMY – it is the total removal of the involved lobe of the lung. This is indicated when the lung lesion is confined to one lobe of the lung. Otherwise, resection of the whole lung does not increase survival.

MASTOIDECTOMY – removal of the bony prominence at the back of the ear through proper debridement of the area by chiseling the pus-filled bones spaces. The patient is put under general anesthesia.

MILES RESECTION – complete removal of the lower portion of the large intestines including the anus. This is done in cases where the tumor or cancer is very near the anal area and reattachment of remaining colon to the anus could not be done. The patient permanently moves his bowel through a **COLOSTOMY** – the proximal portion of the remaining large intestine brought out thru a wound on the left side of the abdomen and a bag collects the feces.

MYOMECTOMY – enucleation or removal of the myoma inside its shell without removal of the uterus.

NEPHROLITHOTOMY - an opening is made on flank whichever side is involved extending from the back down to the flank. The kidney is opened via the CALYSIS and the stone is extracted. Some stones cannot be removed due to its size (STAGHORN) and are therefore crushed prior to removal.

OPEN CYSTOLITHOTOMY – surgical incision done at the lower portion of the abdomen. Urinary catheter is inserted to drain out possible bleeding at the incision.

PACKING OF THE NOSE – strips of gauze bandage is inserted into the nose.

PANENDOSCOPIC LITHOTRIPSY– an instrument is inserted through the penis and crushing probe is used to break the stone to small sizes.

PARENTERAL ANTIBIOTICS – patient has to be admitted for administration of potent antibiotics specific to the kind of bacteria present. This may be in the form of third generation cephalosporin, amino glycosides, and third

PHYSIOTHERAPY – series of exercises to bring back function.

PLATELET CONCENTRATE – transfused to the patient in the event where platelet count drops down below 30,000.

POSTCHOANAL PACKING - a pack of gauze is inserted through the mouth and packed just at the back of the nose above the pharynx.

PYELOLITHOTOMY– it is the removal of stone in the kidney. A large wound is made on the side of the patient extending from the back to the front. The kidney is split open and the stone is removed in toto. 10-15 days stay in the hospital. A 2 to 4 months recovery period is required.

SUTURING OF THE WOUND – wounds if they are more than 2 cm, should be sutured back for cosmetic purposes.

TETANUS TOXOID 1 AMP IM – for tetanus coverage 30 days after bite and the only one given for patients who have complete vaccination prior to the bite/ this will serve as a booster dose.

TETANUS TOXOID VACCINE – for those who have no immunization or immunization was done more than 5 years ago.

THORACENTESIS – insertion of a long needle into the lungs via the 5th – 7th rib space at the back and aspiration of the fluid by a large syringe.

THORACOTOMY – opening of the chest cavity and looking for the bleeding points as seen in chest x-ray. This is a very radical procedure. Anesthesia of the patient is very difficult.

TOTAL ABDOMINAL HYSTERECTOMY – OOPHORECTOMY (TABSHO) – it is the removal of the entire uterus including the ovaries and fallopian tubes. This can be done thru the vagina (TRANS VAGINAL TABSHO) or by opening the abdomen (TRANSABDOMINAL TABSHO).

TOTAL HEPATECTOMY – total removal of the liver. This is followed by liver transplant. Most of these operations are a failure and are considered to be experimental because of frequent rejection.

TOTAL LARYNGECTOMY – total removal of the voice box by surgery. A hole is made at the base of the neck where the distal remaining tube of the lungs (bronchus) is attached and where the patients will now breathe (TRACHEOSTOMY).

TOTAL LOBECTOMY - removal of the entire lung or a lobe of the lung on one side through an opening of the chest called *THORACOTOMY*. Lung capacity of the remaining lung is often measured prior to surgery to determine whether it can support patient post-surgery. Patients with lung impairment like Bronchial asthma, Emphysema, Chronic obstructive lung disease aside from lung cancer would not benefit from this surgery. He would become a LUNG CRIPPLE and would need VENTILATING MACHINE to support him the rest of his days. This surgery may prolong his life 4-6 months more.

T-TUBE CHOLEDOCOSTOMY – inserting a tube into the common bile duct and draining it out through a small skin incision.

URETERAL LITHOTRIPSY – shock waves pointed at the location of the stone, which grinds the stone into fine sand and passed out thru urination.

INDEX

A

ABDOMINAL HYSTERECTOMY 30, 234, 300

ABDOMINAL PAIN 2, 3, 14, 16, 17, 25, 27, 34, 90, 188, 196, 204, 226, 227, 272, 290

ABDOMINAL WALL DEFECT 32, 297

ABRASIONS 87

ABSCESS 89, 123, 124, 128, 135, 136, 140, 141, 152, 153, 154, 155, 156, 229, 248

ACID FAST BACILLI 176, 195, 250, 289

ACUPUNCTURE 84, 104, 106

ACUTE ABDOMEN 9, 28, 296

ACUTE CHOLANGITIS 204

ACUTE CHOLECYSTITIS – CHOLELITHIASIS 16

ACUTE EPIDIDYMITIS 39

ACUTE HOARSENESS 114

ACUTE MASTITIS 53

ACUTE MENINGITIS 72

ACUTE ORCHITIS 76

ACUTE SINUSITIS 62

ACUTE TENDINITIS 80

ACUTE TONSILLITIS 117

ACUTE TYPHOID FEVER 196

ADHESIONS 9

ADJUVANT 6

AFTER MINOR OPERATION 282

AFTERNOON FEVER 175, 194, 251

ALLERGIES 62, 239

ALLERGY 35, 63, 133

AMOEBA 11, 289

ANAL 24, 86, 87, 88, 89, 90, 92, 93, 94, 187, 191, 272, 284, 294, 295, 298,

ANAL CANAL 94, 187, 191, 294, 295

ANAL CREAMS 93

ANAL PAIN IN HEMORRHOIDS 92

ANAL PAINS 86, 87

ANAL SUPPOSITORY 93

ANALGESICS 51, 52, 61, 63, 65, 66, 81, 82, 84, 89, 93, 97, 104, 106, 129, 135, 136, 137, 148, 160, 163, 213, 280, 282

ANGINA 11

ANTI – HYPERTENSIVE 69, 211

ANTI – TB DRUGS 49, 102

302

ANTI –INFLAMMATORY 93

ANTIBIOTICS.... 10, 28, 39, 49, 50, 63, 73, 89, 108, 109, 112, 113, 114, 115, 118, 129, 131, 135, 136, 138, 148, 152, 155, 158, 160, 162, 204, 238, 239, 280, 282, 286, 299

APPENDECTOMY 8, 9, 169, 293, 296

APPENDICITIS 3, 7, 8, 9, 189, 285, 296

APPENDIX.. 7, 8, 291, 293

ARTHRITIS 47, 68, 78, 284

ASO TITER 113, 284

ASPIRATION OF THE FLUID... 49, 299

ASYMPTOMATIC 158, 166

B

BACK PAIN + COUGH +SMOKING 99

BACK PAIN + HISTORY OF TB 101

BACK PAINS 101, 103, 104, 105, 194

BARIUM ENEMA... 24, 26, 91, 189, 227, 284

BASAL CELL CARCINOMA 240

BETAMETHASONE INTRATHECAL INJECTION 81, 293

*BIOPSY*4, 6, 51, 55, 56, 57, 58, 59, 60, 91, 94, 116, 119, 172, 173, 175, 177, 223, 224, 225, 227, 229, 230, 231, 234, 235, 238, 240, 245, 252, 254, 282, 284, 285, 286, 287, 288, 289, 295, 296

BLEEDING 9, 29, 30, 87, 90, 91, 94, 129, 130, 145, 148, 151, 161, 162, 163, 164, 171, 172, 174, 175, 178, 179, 180, 181, 182, 183, 184, 185, 186, 187, 188, 189, 190, 191, 217, 234, 258, 272, 274, 277, 278, 287, 289, 293, 295, 299, 300

BLOOD IN ANUS AND STOOLS.. 186

BLOOD IN THE SPUTUM.. 174, 231

BLOOD IN URINE 164

BLOOD POISONING 8

BLOOD URIC.. 47, 284

BLOOD VOMIT.. 181

BLOODY SPUTUM + COUGH + AFTERNOON FEVER.. 175

BLOODY SPUTUM + LOST OF WEIGHT + CHEST PAINS 176

BLOODY SPUTUM + SEVERE FORCEFUL COUGH 178

BLOODY URINE + FREQUENCY OF URINATION... 170

BLOODY URINE + NO URINARY STREAM FORCE 172

BLOODY URINE + PAIN INGUINAL AND SCROTUM (MALE).. 168

BLUNTING OF THE COSTOPHRENIC ANGLE 49

BONE JOINTS.. 78

BRAIN 61, 65, 66, 72, 73, 145, 185, 209, 210, 211, 212, 213, 235, 236, 240, 242, 257, 274, 286, 288

BRAIN TUMOR 65, 209, 213, 235

BREAST INDURATIONS 55

BREAST PAIN + A MASS IN AN 18 YR OLD 55

BREAST PAIN + MASS IN A 35 YR OLD 57

BREAST PAIN + NIPPLE DISCHARGE (BLOODY) IN A 25 YR OLD 59

BREAST PAIN + ROUND MASS IN A 21 YR OLD 56

BREAST PAIN DURING LACTATION 53

BREAST PAIN DURING MENOPAUSE 54

BRONCHOSCOPY 100, 116, 121, 177, 178, 179, 284, 288, 293

BRONCHUS 113, 117, 120, 121, 162, 177, 178, 200, 216, 284, 293, 296, 300

BURNS 279, 280

C

CALCIUM 35, 95, 99, 243

CALISTHENICS 82, 84, 104

CANCER ... 5, 17, 18, 20, 23, 24, 49, 52, 57, 58, 99, 100, 116, 119, 127, 172, 175, 176, 177, 181, 203, 222, 223, 224, 225, 226, 227, 228, 229, 230, 231, 234, 235, 237, 238, 239, 240, 242, 243, 245, 246, 251, 252, 253, 284, 286, 288, 289, 290, 294, 297, 298, 300

CANCER OF THE LIVER 18, 229, 230, 305

CANCER OF THE LUNGS 99, 231, 252

CAT BITE 143

CATARACT. 70, 264

CEREBRAL CONCUSSION / CEREBRAL HEMATOMA 212

CEREBRO-SPINAL FLUID 73, 288

CERVICAL SPONDYLITIS 82

CHEMOTHERAPY 6, 20, 49, 100, 117, 142, 173, 177, 255, 228, 230, 238, 240

CHEST PAIN 11, 43, 44, 45, 46, 47, 50, 176, 205, 225

CHEST PAINS + HYPERACIDITY 45

CHEST TUBE INSERTION 49, 158, 293

CHEST X- RAY 13, 49

CHILLS 14, 21, 195, 204

CHOKING 119, 277, 280

CHOLECYSTITIS 16, 17

CHOLESTEROL 12, 16, 35, 70, 256, 288

CHRONIC HOARSENESS 116

COBALT TREATMENT 117, 294

COIL SIGN

   INTUSSUSCEPTION 25, 26

COLD SHOWERS 65

COLDS 112, 113, 114, 115, 116, 117, 200, 258

COLON.. 24, 90, 91, 160, 188, 298

COLONIC CANCER.. 23

COLONOSCOPY.. 24, 88, 91, 186, 189, 227, 285

COLOSTOMY 24, 91, 228, 297, 298

COMMON COLD... 62, 115

COMPLETE BLOOD COUNT... 8, 28, 148, 201, 285

COMPLETE JOINT REPLACEMENT... 79, 294

CONGENITAL 33, 246

CONGESTIVE HEART FAILURE.. 49, 257

CONSTIPATION... 23, 25, 87, 90, 92, 189, 191, 227, 258

CONTUSION 129

CONVULSION 211, 276, 279

CORONARY ANGIOGRAM.. 12, 285

CORONARY BYPASS.. 13, 294

CORONARY STENT.. 13, 294

COUGH.. 48, 96, 99, 101, 112, 113, 114, 115, 174, 175, 178, 194, 200, 205, 206, 251, 258, 279, 280

CT SCAN 5, 8, 12, 15, 17, 20, 26, 28, 32, 65, 67, 73, 83, 85, 91, 100, 102, 104, 106, 117, 160, 162, 167, 177, 179, 185, 211, 212, 214, 230, 231, 235, 238, 245, 254, 286

CULTURE AND SENSITIVITY 22, 113, 136, 138, 249, 186

CYSTS 140, 222, 223, 229, 238, 239, 242

CYSTS AND CANCER 222, 223, 238

D

DARK DISCOLORATION OF THE SKIN 141

DECONGESTANTS.. 63, 114

DIABETES MELLITUS..12, 155, 261

DIABETIC 239, 262, 264, 277

DIABETIC GANGRENE 262

DIAMOND TECHNIQUE 94, 191, 295

DIFFICULTY OF BREATHING.......................... 42, 43, 48, 114, 120, 133, 146, 158, 162, 184, 205, 218, 219, 268, 296

DIFFICULTY OF SWALLOWING..117, 119, 226, 238, 253

DIFFICULTY OF SWALLOWING + FEVER 117

DIFFICULTY OF SWALLOWING + NO FEVER 119

DIRECT INHALATION 175

TUBERCULOSIS OF THE LUNGS..174, 175, 194, 250

305

DIVERTICULUM 188, 189

DRAINAGE OF THE SINUSES 64, 295, 297

DROPS OF BLOOD IN THE TOILET BOWL 190

DROWNING..64, 278, 295

DRUNK 277

DRUNK SEVERE VOMITING BLOOD 182

DYSMENORRHEA 32

DYSPNEA 31, 219

E

ECG (ELECTROCARDIOGRAM) 12, 47, 286

ELECTRICAL BURNS 280

ENLARGEMENT OF THE NECK 241, 242, 243

EPIDERMOID CYST 239

EPIGASTRIC PAIN.. 3, 4, 5, 7, 9, 11, 13, 44

EPIGASTRIC PAIN + RIGHT OF LEFT FLANK PAIN 13

EPIGASTRIC PAINS + NONHEALING ULCER 5

EPIGASTRIC PAINS + RIGHT LOWER QUADRANT PAIN 7

ERROR OF REFRACTION 70

ERYTHEMA 134, 146, 250

ESOPHAGEAL CANCER.. 119, 253

ESOPHAGOSCOPY 182, 183, 287, 295

ESOPHAGUS 42, 45, 119, 120, 121, 125, 181, 182, 183, 226, 227, 228, 238, 253, 254, 287, 295

ESTROGEN...51, 52, 54, 55, 229

EXCISIONAL BIOPSY 57, 58, 60, 224, 252, 295

EXPLORATORY LAPAROTOMY 9, 26, 28, 160, 205, 296

EYE CATARACT 264

EYE STRAIN.. 70

F

FASTING BLOOD SUGAR...142, 155, 261, 287

FECAL CHARACTERISTICS 272

FEVER.3, 7, 14, 18, 21, 26, 38, 72, 74, 75, 76, 112, 113, 114, 116, 117, 119, 123, 134, 148, 166, 175, 192, 193, 194, 195, 196, 197, 198, 199, 200, 201, 202, 203, 204, 205, 206, 248, 251, 272, 279, 289

FEVER + COLD + COUGH.. 200

FEVER + COUGH + DIFFICULTY OF BREATHING 205

FEVER + JAUNDICE 204

FEVER + RASHES ON LEGS 198

FEVER + WATERY STOOLS + HEADACHE 196

FEVER + YELLOWISH 202

FEVER WITH CHILLS 195

FIBER – OPTIC 227

FIBROCYSTIC DISEASE OF THE BREAST 56

FINE NEEDLE BIOPSY 57, 58, 224, 230, 231, 245, 287, 296

FISSURES 87, 187

FISTULA IN ANUS 88, 94

FISTULECTOMY 89, 296

FLANK PAIN 13, 34, 164, 195, 196

FLEET ENEMA 23

FRACTURES 47, 77, 130, 131, 158, 162, 216, 217, 279, 291, 292

FREQUENCY OF URINATION 21, 170, 172, 195

FRESH BLOOD FROM THE ANUS 158, 159

FRESH BLOOD IN THE ANUS 186, 187

FRONTAL HEADACHE 62

FROZEN SECTION 57, 224, 297

FUNCTION LAETIA 208, 217

FURUNCULOSIS 137

G

GALL BLADDER 8, 16, 17, 18, 203, 204, 205, 252, 290, 291, 293, 298

GANGLION CYST 239

GASTRECTOMY 6, 227, 297

GASTRIC MALIGNANCY 5

GASTROINTESTINAL TRACT 6, 180, 183, 226, 228, 297

GASTROSCOPY 4, 6, 119, 182, 227, 287, 295

GENERALIZED HEADACHE 72

GLASS 40, 71, 108, 150, 151, 166, 291

GONORRHEA 107

GRAM STAINS OF STOOLS 11, 287

GRAM STAINING OF THROAT 113

GYNECOLOGIST 29

H

H. PYLORI 4, 287

H₂BLOCKERS 5

HEADACHES 61, 63, 66, 67, 72, 196, 197, 213, 235, 256, 258

HEART 11, 12, 13, 42, 43, 44, 45, 46, 47, 49, 112, 113, 245, 257, 263, 268, 270, 274, 275, 278, 284, 285, 286, 294

HEART ATTACK 12, 13, 43, 47, 268, 275, 286

HEARTBURN 45

HEMATOMA 35, 60, 130, 131, 212, 217, 298

HEMICOLECTOMY 24, 91, 227, 297

HEMORRHOIDECTOMY 191

HEMORRHOIDS 87, 89, 90, 92, 94, 187, 188, 190, 191, 272, 284, 295

HEPATITIS B 18, 19, 203, 229, 287

HERPES ZOSTER 50

HISTOPATHOLOGIC DIAGNOSIS 57

HORIZONTAL LACERATIONS 163

HUMAN BITE 148, 149

HYOID BONE 246, 247

HYPERACIDITY 45, 46

HYPERTENSION 69, 70, 185, 209, 210, 255, 256, 257, 258, 259, 284, 288

HYPOCALCEMIA 98

HYPOGASTRIC PAINS + VAGINAL SPOTTING 29

HYPOGASTRIC 7, 9, 21, 29, 30, 164, 296

HYPOGASTRIC PAINS + FREQUENCY OF URINATION 21

HYPOGASTRIC PAINS + MENSTRUATION 30

HYPOGLOSSAL DUCT CYST 246

HYPOGONADISM 54

HYPOPARATHYROIDISM 243, 245

HYPOTHYROIDISM 243, 245

HYSTERECTOMY 30, 234, 297, 300

I

IMPOTENCE AND HYPOSPERMIA 264

IN TESTICULAR TORSION 41

IN THE NECK 13, 110, 111, 161, 245, 277, 294

IN VARICOCELE 40

INCISION AND DRAINAGE 53, 64, 124, 135, 136, 141, 239, 297

INCISION AND DRAINAGE OF THE LATERAL CHAMBERS 64, 297

INFECTED SEBACEOUS CYST 139

INFECTION OF THE KIDNEY 14

INFRA-AURICULAR PAIN 75

INGUINAL HERNIA 32

INGUINAL PAIN 32, 168

INSECT BITE 132, 133, 146,147

INTERSCAPULAR PAINS 96

INTRADUCTAL PAPILLOMA 59

INTRAVENOUS PYELOGRAM 15, 35, 169, 288

INTUSSUSCEPTION 25, 26

IODINE DEFICIENCY 241

ISORDIL SUBLINGUAL 12, 44, 275

ITCHINESS OF THE SKIN 18

J

JOINT PAINS 78, 79

K

KIDNEY 8, 14, 15, 17, 34, 35, 70, 79, 142, 160, 164, 166, 167, 168, 169, 181, 195, 196, 252, 256, 257, 262, 263, 264, 285, 288, 290, 298, 299

KIDNEY – URETER 167

KIDNEY FAILURE 70, 142, 181, 256, 257, 262

KIDNEY STONE 8, 15, 34, 35, 166, 167, 169, 290, 298

KNOTTING OF THE SMALL INTESTINE 27

L

LACERATION................................... 35, 87, 144, 148, 162, 163, 167, 178, 181, 182, 183, 184, 185, 187, 198

LAMINECTOMY 83, 85, 106, 298

LAPAROSCOPE.. 17, 298

LAPAROSCOPIC CHOLECYSTECTOMY 17, 298

LARGE INTESTINE 23, 24, 25, 26, 88, 90, 91, 120, 186, 189, 191, 227, 228, 254, 285, 289, 294, 295, 297, 298

LARYNGEAL BIOPSY OF THE TUMOR 116, 288

LARYNGEAL TUMOR.. 116

LARYNX 114, 115, 116, 238

LAXATIVES..87, 93, 187

LEFT LOWER QUADRANT PAIN IN THE ADULT 23

LEFT LOWER QUADRANT PAIN IN THE YOUNG 25

LEGS AND TOES OF A SMOKER... 270

LIPID PROFILE 70, 288

LIPOMA 239

LIVER 17, 18, 19, 20, 23, 26, 65, 79, 127, 141, 142, 160, 175, 181, 202, 203, 204, 229, 230, 240, 251, 252, 269, 270, 284, 286, 287, 289, 290, 297, 298, 300

LIVER OF THE SMOKER 269

LOBECTOMY 20, 100, 177, 230, 232, 297, 298, 300

LOSS OF CONSCIOUSNESS 11, 61, 66, 213, 274

LOW BACK PAINS 103, 105

LOW BACK PAINS + SHOOTING PAINS TO THE LEGS 105

LUMBAGO 103

LUMBAR SPONDYLITIS 84, 103

LUMBAR TAP... 73, 288

LUNGS 13, 42, 48, 49, 99, 100, 102, 113, 117, 121, 158, 174, 175, 176, 177, 178, 180, 194, 205, 206, 216, 231, 232, 240, 250, 251, 252, 257, 267, 269, 270, 284, 285, 286, 293, 299, 300

LYMPH NODES 134, 148, 225, 246, 248, 250

M

MALIGNANCY 4, 5, 54, 55, 56, 57, 59, 94, 120, 125, 189, 191, 214, 243, 284, 287, 294, 297

MAMMOGRAPHY 51, 52, 55, 56, 223, 224, 252, 288

MANTOUX 250

MASS ABOVE THE ADAM'S APPLE 246

MASS BASE OF THE NECK 251

MASS IN THE ANTERIOR NECK 244

MASS ON THE SIDE OF THE NECK 253

MASS UNDER THE MANDIBLE 248

MASTOID 74, 298

MELANOMA 240

MENINGES 72, 73

MENOPAUSAL SYNDROME 54

MENSTRUATION 30, 31, 51, 52, 54, 56, 233

MENTHOL LINIMENTS 63

MIGRAINE HEADACHE 64, 235

MILES RESECTION 24, 91, 228, 298

MODIFIED RADICAL NECK DISSECTION 246
MOLE 240
MRI 5, 79, 81, 83, 85, 104, 106, 216, 288
MUCOID BLOOD... 25, 272
MUMPS..38, 39, 75
MUSCLE RELAXANT 98
MYALGIA 96
MYCOBACTERIUM TUBERCULOSIS..101, 175, 194
MYOCARDIAL INFARCTION 11
MYOMA 29, 30, 234, 298
MYOMECTOMY... 30, 298

N

NAUSEA 3, 5, 7, 9, 25, 30, 66, 72, 183, 258
NECROSIS 41, 154, 156, 234
NERVES FOUND IN THE SCALP 64
NITRITES... 12
NON – GONOCOCCAL URETHRITIS 109
NON – MALIGNANT 55
NONHEALING ULCER... 5
NORMAL LUNG 267
NOSE BLEEDING 184, 185
NUCHAL PAIN..69, 211, 256
NUMBNESS OF LEFT ARM 43

O

OCCIPITAL PAIN... 70
ON THE ABDOMEN 7, 26, 30, 169, 183, 278, 295
ON THE CHEST BUT NOT MUCH BLEEDING.. 278
ON THE CHEST WITH SPURTING BLOOD 278
ON THE HEAD.. 212, 277
ON THE THIGHS AND ARMS 278
OSTEOARTHRITIS 78

P

PAIN ..2, 3, 4, 5, 6, 7, 9, 10, 11, 13, 14, 15, 16, 17, 18, 19, 21, 23, 25, 27, 29, 30, 31, 32, 34, 35, 36, 37, 38, 40, 41, 42, 43, 44, 45, 46, 47, 48, 50, 51, 52, 53, 54, 55, 56, 57, 59, 61, 62, 65, 66, 67, 68, 69, 70, 72, 74, 75, 77, 78, 79, 80, 81, 82, 84, 86, 87, 88, 89, 90, 91, 92, 94, 95, 96, 97, 98, 99, 101, 103, 104, 105, 107, 109, 110, 111, 112, 113, 114, 117, 118, 119, 122, 123, 124, 130, 133, 134, 139, 141, 146, 152, 153, 154, 164, 166, 167, 168, 169, 170, 172, 176, 187, 188, 194, 195, 196, 200, 204, 205, 208, 211, 217, 223, 225, 226, 227, 231, 233, 239, 244, 247, 248, 256, 264, 270, 272, 279, 282, 283, 289, 290, 293, 294, 298

PAIN AND NUMBNESS OF THE UPPER EXTREMITY 82
PAIN AT THE ANAL SIDE 88
PAIN DURING URINATION 21, 107, 109, 166, 170, 195
PAIN DURING URINATION WITHOUT DISCHARGE 109
PAIN IN THE EAR 122, 123, 124
PAIN IN THE EAR + FULLNESS 123
PAIN IN THE EAR + ITCHINESS 124
PAIN IN THE NECK DURING SWALLOWING 110
PAIN IN THE SCROTUM 38, 40, 41, 290
PAIN ON INSPIRATION 46
PAINS OF THE CHEST AND BREAST PAINS 42
PALPITATIONS 64, 256
PAPILLOMA 59, 60, 239
PARALYSIS 61, 72, 209, 210, 212, 213, 214, 216, 235, 257, 294
PARALYSIS AFTER BACK BONE INJURY 214
PARALYSIS DUE TO BRAIN TUMOR 213
PARALYSIS DUE TO STROKE 210
PARALYSIS DUE TO TRAUMA TO THE HEAD 212
PARASITISM 11, 289
PARATHYROID HORMONE 245
PARENTERAL ANTIBIOTICS 73, 299
PAROTID GLAND 75, 82
PAST PHYSICAL TRAUMA 65
PELVIC INFLAMMATORY DISEASE 189
PENILE 14, 40, 107, 108, 109, 173, 286, 291
PENIS 107, 109, 171, 299
PEPTIC ULCER 4, 46, 272, 287
PERIPHERAL NEUROPATHY 264
PLATELET COUNT 181, 185, 199, 289, 299
PLEURAL EFFUSION 48, 49
PNEUMOTHORAX.. 158, 293

POSTAURICULAR PAIN 74

PREVIOUS PSYCHOLOGICAL TRAUMA 65

PROCTOSIGMOIDOSCOPY 88, 91, 187, 191, 289

PUS 8, 9, 15, 53, 74, 88, 135, 136, 137, 138, 141, 153, 154, 155, 156, 196, 225, 262, 291, 293, 295, 298

PYELOLITHOTOMY 35, 299

R

RADIATION OF THE NECK 246

RADIOACTIVE IODINE UPTAKE 242

RAIU 242

RAT BITE 147, 148

RECTAL EXAMINATION 89, 90, 186, 289

REDDENING AND DARK 128

REDDENING OF THE SKIN 128, 129, 130, 134, 135, 143, 146, 147

REFLUX ESOPHAGUS – HEARTBURN 45

RIGID SCOPE 88, 289

RIBS 47, 49, 158, 293

RIGHT INGUINAL PAIN (OR LEFT) + MASS IN THE SCROTUM 32

RIGHT LOWER QUADRANT PAIN 7

RIGHT OR LEFT FLANK PAIN 13, 34

RIGHT UPPER QUADRANT PAIN 16, 18

ROWING 80, 136

RULE OUT MALIGNANCY 57

S

SCIATICA SECONDARY TO LUMBAR SPONDYLITIS 84

SCROTAL PAINS 36

SCROTUM 32, 33, 34, 36, 38, 39, 40, 41, 164, 168, 290

SEBACEOUS CYST 139, 140, 238, 239

SEPTICEMIA 8

SERUM CALCIUM DETERMINATION 99

SEXUALLY TRANSMITTED DISEASE 21, 36, 39, 109

SIGMOID 189

SINUSES 62, 63, 64, 73, 295, 297

SKIN. 8, 18, 50, 54, 87, 89, 91, 102, 128, 129, 130, 131, 132, 133, 134, 135, 136, 137, 139, 141, 142, 143, 146, 147, 152, 153, 154, 155, 156, 163, 175, 204, 205, 225, 238, 239, 240, 241, 250, 261, 262, 269, 270, 277, 279, 280, 290, 293, 300

SKIN ABSCESS WITH PUSTULE 154

SKIN ABSCESS WITHOUT OPENING 152

SKIN INFECTION 134, 261

SKIN TAGS 240

SKIN ULCERATION 155, 156

SMALL INTESTINE 6, 10, 27, 196, 205, 226, 227, 228, 294, 297

SMOKER'S LUNG 268

SMOKING 99, 100, 176, 177, 178, 231, 252, 265, 266, 267, 268, 270

SONOGRAM 51, 52, 55, 284

SORE THROAT 112, 113, 114, 116, 117, 238, 248, 284

SORE THROAT + ACUTE HOARSENESS 114

SORE THROAT + CHRONIC HOARSENESS 116

SORE THROAT + COLDS 113

SPINAL CORD 83, 102, 104, 105, 106, 214, 215, 216, 288, 291

SPINE 101, 102

SPONTANEOUS NOSE BLEEDING 184, 185

SQUAMOUS CANCER 240

STABBED WOUNDS AND GUN SHOT WOUNDS 277

STAPHYLOCOCCUS 136, 137

STERILITY 38, 40, 76

STOMACH 4, 5, 6, 17, 42, 45, 79, 119, 120, 121, 160, 182, 183, 186, 205, 226, 227, 228, 251, 253, 254, 284, 287, 293, 294, 295, 297

STOOL CHARACTERISTICS IN LOOSE BOWEL MOVEMENT 271, 272

STOOL EXAM 11, 289

STREPTOCOCCAL INFECTION 112, 315

STRESS 4, 12, 44, 45, 66, 67, 99, 101, 103, 179

STRESS HEADACHE 66

STRESS PAINS 66

STROKE 209, 210, 211, 257

SUPERFICIAL WOUND 150, 158

SURGERY ..6, 8, 9, 17, 26, 28, 30, 32, 33, 41, 46, 51, 71, 79, 83, 89, 94, 100, 102, 106, 116, 117, 118, 119, 135, 136, 153, 158, 167, 169, 173, 177, 182, 183, 191, 204, 205, 214, 216, 217, 224, 227, 228, 236, 239, 242, 245, 246, 247, 264, 272, 285, 286, 292, 293, 294, 295, 296, 300

SWALLOWED COINS 120

T

TENNIS ELBOW 80, 81

TESTICULAR TORSION 41

THERAPEUTIC 26, 178, 183, 287

THYROID 242, 243, 244, 245, 246

THYROID TUMOR 244

THYROIDECTOMY 243, 245, 246

THYROXINE 242

TONSILS AND PHARYNX 112, 180

TORSION 41, 215

TORTICULIS 98

TOTAL LARYNGECTOMY 117, 300

TOXIC GOITER 241, 242

TRAUMATIZED NOSE BLEEDING 185

TREAD MILL 12

TSH 242

TUBERCULOSIS OF THE SPINE 101

TUMORS AND CANCERS OF THE INTESTINE 226

TUMORS OF THE BRAIN 213, 235

TUMORS OF THE LIVER 229, 230

TWISTED OVARIAN CYST 189

TYPHOID 11, 196, 197, 291

U

ULCER 4, 5, 6, 46, 138, 146, 148, 155, 156, 225, 239, 240, 262, 272, 287

ULTRASOUND 5, 8, 12, 15, 17, 20, 26, 28, 31, 32, 35, 38, 40, 160, 167, 169, 171, 172, 203, 204, 223, 230, 234, 235, 242, 245, 247, 252, 290, 291

ULTRASOUND (2D ECHOCARDIOGRAM) 12

ULTRASOUND OF THE ABDOMEN 26

ULTRASOUND OF THE GALL BLADDER 17, 290

ULTRASOUND OF THE SCROTUM 38, 40, 290

UPPER GI SERIES 4, 6, 227, 290

UPPER RESPIRATORY 8, 73, 115, 200, 201, 206, 285

UPRIGHT FILM OF THE ABDOMEN 26, 28, 160, 291

URETER 15, 34, 35, 164, 166, 167, 168, 169, 288, 290, 300

URETEROLITHOTOMY 35, 169

URETHRA.. 14, 22, 40, 108, 109, 164, 291

URETHRAL SMEAR ...., 40, 108, 109, 291

URIC ACID DETERMINATION 47, 79, 284

URINALYSIS 8, 14, 15, 22, 35, 38, 39, 40, 108, 109, 165, 167, 169, 171, 172, 196, 261, 291

URINARY BLADDER 14, 15, 21, 35, 164, 166, 167, 168, 169, 170, 171, 189, 195, 233, 288, 290, 296
URINARY TRACT INFECTION 8, 14, 21, 37, 39, 108, 109, 164, 195
UTERINE MYOMA... 29
UTERUS 29, 30, 31, 32, 233, 234, 289, 290, 297, 298, 300
UTI 22, 39, 40,

V

VAGINAL HYSTERECTOMY... 30, 297
VARICOCELE 40
VERTICAL LACERATIONS.. 163
VESICLE FORMATION 50
VIRAL INFECTION 50, 75, 82, 113, 114, 198, 200, 201, 202
VISUAL DEFECT 70
VOLVULUS... 27
VOMITING BLOOD (HEMATEMESIS) 180

W

WARM WATER SHOWERS... 63
WET ANUS.. 94, 191
WHITEHEAD TECHNIQUE 94
WOUND CARE 281
WOUNDS............................... 126, 127, 148, 149, 150, 157, 158, 159, 161, 162, 163, 217, 277, 280, 295, 299
WOUNDS AND BLUNT INJURY TO THE ABDOMEN... 159
WOUNDS OF THE FACE 163

X

X- RAY OF THE ABDOMEN... 8
X-RAY OF THE JOINT... 79, 81
X-RAY OF THE LUMBAR VERTEBRAE 85, 106
X-RAY OF THE MANDIBLE.. 68
X-RAYS.............................. 24, 89, 130, 158, 167, 175, 189, 216, 217, 223, 227, 235, 284, 288, 291

Y

YELLOW DISCOLORATION OF THE EYES 18

THE AUTHOR

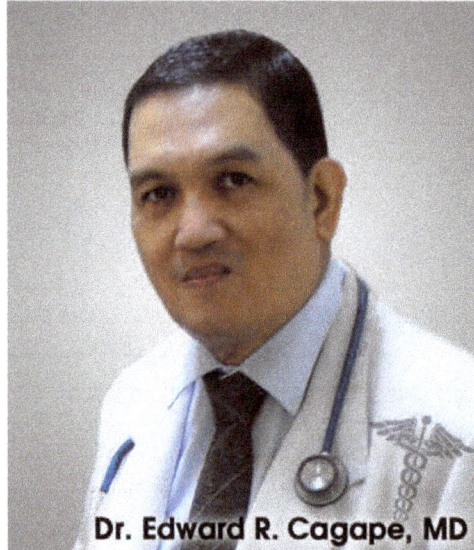

Dr. Edward R. Cagape, MD

Having a background in humanities and being exposed to patients from all walks in life, Dr. Edward Cagape is a general surgeon who is concerned regarding the overall well-being of his patients. As such, his concern extends to the emotional, psychosocial and spiritual state.

Dr. Cagape is a product of Univeristy of Sto. Tomas where he earned his Doctorate degree after taking Bachelor of Science in Natural Sciences in Ateneo de Davao. He specializes in thyroid, breast and gastrointestinal tract and has established a Cyst Center in Davao City. Although he practices general surgery, it did not keep him from being consulted on different types of body ailments. He is happy to be called as "everyone's physician".

Not just an ordinary physician, Dr. Cagape has remarkable achievements: he became a Medical Director of Coca-Cola Bottlers Philippines-Mindanao and clinical instructor of Davao Medical School Foundation, he was the Chief Resident Physician of the Davao Doctors Hospital, and a Medical Consultant of ABS-CBN's Lingkod Bayan Program.

But, there is more to Dr. Cagape than surgery as he became a medical columnist in Mindanao Daily Mirror. He is a natural charmer due to his essentially human approach towards his patients. Hence, he earned the distinction of being the "Patch Adams" of Davao. Showing his versatility in media, he also hosted the University of Mindanao Broadcasting Network program called Doctor on the Air (Doktor sa Kahanginan). His daily prime time radio enlightened listeners as he discussed medicine, sickness and overall health in layman's term. Just like the real Patch Adam, Dr. Cagape shows his passion towards his work through his wit and humor.